Alfons G. Hofstetter (Ed.)
Lasers in Urological Surgery

Springer

Berlin
Heidelberg
New York
Barcelona
Budapest
Hong Kong
London
Milan
Paris
Santa Clara
Singapore
Tokyo

ALFONS G. HOFSTETTER (Ed.)

Lasers in Urological Surgery

With Contributions by
R. Baumgartner · H.-P. Berlien · A. Ehsan · F. Frank
A. Friesen · B. Fuchs · W. Gorisch · A. G. Hofstetter
R. Klammert · M. Kriegmair · W. Lubos · G. Müller
R. Muschter · K.-H. Rothenberger · N. Schmeller
P. Schneede · W. Waidelich · F. Wondrazek

With 92 Figures, Some in Color

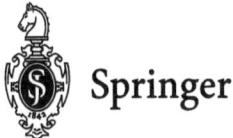 Springer

Alfons G. Hofstetter, M.D.
Professor of Urology, Director and Chairman
Urologische Klinik und Poliklinik
Klinikum Grosshadern und Innenstadt
Ludwig-Maximilians-Universität
Marchioninistrasse 15
81377 München, Germany

Title of the German Edition:
A. G. Hofstetter (Hrsg.), Laser in der Urologie
© Springer-Verlag Berlin Heidelberg 1995

ISBN-13: 978-3-642-95837-3

Cip data applied for.

Die Deutsche Bibliothek – CIP-Einheitsaufnahme
Lasers in urological surgery/Alfons G. Hofstetter (ed.). With contribu-
tions by R. Baumgartner... – Berlin; Heidelberg; New York; Barcelona;
Budapest; Hong Kong; London; Milan; Paris; Santa Clara; Singapore;
Tokyo: Springer, 1997.
Dt. Ausgabe u.d.T.: Laser in der Urologie
ISBN-13: 978-3-642-95837-3   e-ISBN-13: 978-3-642-95835-9
DOI: 10.1007/978-3-642-95835-9

English Translation: Terry C. Telger, Fort Worth, TX, USA

Typesetting: Mitterweger Werksatz GmbH, 68723 Plankstadt, Germany

SPIN 10552978   13/3135   5 4 3 2 1 0 – Printed on acid-free paper

Preface

The introduction of lasers into operative medicine and advances in fiberoptic technology have made a significant contribution to minimally invasive surgery. This book was written to raise awareness of the capabilities and advantages of lasers in urological surgery and to make this technology more widely accessible. The book reflects the cumulative experience of 25 years of laser research and clinical application, starting in 1972 with studies on laser-tissue interactions, endoscopic studies with fiberoptic "sutures," and the first clinical use of lasers in 1975 and 1976. These early efforts were followed by the development of laser lithotripsy in the early 1980 s and a Lubeck-based research program leading to the development of a "smart" laser lithotriptor (Lithognost) in the late 1980s.

There have been recent advances in the field of photodynamic diagnosis based on the use of locally administered photosensitizers, a development that will redefine the role of the Nd:YAG laser in the treatment of bladder cancer. Perhaps the most interesting concept is the interstitial laser therapy of prostatic hyperplasia and, perhaps one day, certain forms of prostatic cancer. We have also developed a technique, first described in 1986, for the laser treatment of schistosomal bladder lesions.

I dedicate this book to the many pioneers of laser medicine and to all the colleagues and research assistants who accompanied me on this journey. I cannot name them all; their names can be found in more than 300 publications. But I will list the pioneers whom I, as the president of the German Society for Laser Medicine, have been privileged to induct as honorary members and who have supported my research throughout the years. These are:

B. Antoni (Hungary) †, P. Ascher (Austria), J. Atsumi (Japan), G. Banhidy (Hungary), B. Benson (United States), K. Dinstl (Austria), L. Fischer (Austria) †, F. Frank (Germany), F. Heppner (Austria), J. Kaplan (Israel), E. Keiditsch (Germany), P. Kiefhaber (Germany), H. Müssiggang (Germany), T. Maiman (United States), T. Malloy

(United States), J. Prokohov (USSR), K.-H. Rothenberger (Germany), E. Schmiedt (Germany), O. Schmidt (Hungary), A. Shanberg (United States), J. Smith (United States), G. Staehler (Germany), R. Skobelkin (USSR), Van Gemert (Netherlands), G. Wabrosch (Hungary), W. Waidelich (Germany).

I wish to thank all those who contributed to this book, which I hope will help pave the way for a new surgical modality. I also thank Springer Verlag for the high production quality of this book, with special thanks to Dr. Bacchus and Dr. Heilmann for their enthusiasm for the project and their willingness to help whenever and wherever necessary to see the book to its completion.

Munich, April 1997   A.G. HOFSTETTER

Contents

Theoretical Principles 1

1   Laser Physics 3
    W. WAIDELICH

2   Safety Aspects of Laser Surgery 27
    F. FRANK and F. WONDRAZEK

3   User Certification, Equipment Safety,
    and Laser Safety Officer 39
    B. FUCHS, H.-P. BERLIEN, G. MÜLLER,
    and W. GORISCH

Clinical Laser Use 45

4   Thermal Effects of Lasers 47

4.1   External Genitalia 47
4.1.1 Condylomata Acuminata
      and Other Viral Skin Lesions 47
      P. SCHNEEDE and A.G. HOFSTETTER
4.1.2 Penile Carcinoma 56
      K.-H. ROTHENBERGER and A.G. HOFSTETTER

4.2   Urethra 62
4.2.1 Laser Treatment of Urethral Strictures 62
      P. SCHNEEDE, R. KLAMMERT,
      and A.G. HOFSTETTER

4.3   Bladder 67
      A.G. HOFSTETTER
4.3.1 Bladder Cancer 67
4.3.2 Urinary Schistosomiasis 77
4.3.3 Interstitial Cystitis
      (Hunner's Ulcer, Submucous Fibrosis) 81

4.4   Ureter 83
        A.G. HOFSTETTER
4.4.1   Ureteral Tumors 83

4.5   Pyelocaliceal System 88
        A.G. HOFSTETTER
4.5.1   Pyelocaliceal Tumors 88

4.6   Laparoscopic Pelvic Lymphadenectomy 93
        W. LUBOS, N. SCHMELLER,
        and A.G. HOFSTETTER

4.7   Laser-Assisted Vasovasostomy 100
        A. FRIESEN

4.8   Prostate 102
        R. MUSCHTER and A.G. HOFSTETTER
4.8.1   Benign Prostatic Hyperplasia 103
4.8.2   Prostatic Carcinoma 114

5   Photodynamic Diagnosis and Therapy
        of Superficial Bladder Cancer 119
        M. KRIEGMAIR, R. BAUMGARTNER,
        and A.G. HOFSTETTER

5.1   Theoretical Principles 119
5.2   Photodynamic Diagnosis 121
5.3   Photodynamic Therapy 124

6   Laser Lithotripsy of Ureteral Stones 131
        A.G. HOFSTETTER, N. SCHMELLER,
        and A. EHSAN

7   Future Prospects 137
        A.G. HOFSTETTER

Appendix 139

        Instrumentation 141

Subject Index 151

Contributors

BAUMGARTNER, R., Dr. rer. nat.
Urologische Universitätsklinik, Klinikum Grosshadern
Marchioninistrasse 15, 81377 München, Germany

BERLIEN, H.-P., Professor Dr. med.
Fachgebiet Lasermedizin, Klinikum Steglitz
Freie Universität Berlin
Hindenburgdamm 30, 12203 Berlin, Germany

EHSAN, A., Dr. med.
Urologische Universitätsklinik, Klinikum Grosshadern
Marchioninistrasse 15, 81377 München, Germany

FRANK, F., Dr. rer. nat.
Sarreiter Weg 13, 85560 Ebersberg, Germany

FRIESEN, A., Dr. med.
Urologische Abteilung
Städtisches Krankenhaus, München-Bogenhausen
Englschalkingerstrasse 77, 81925 München, Germany

FUCHS, B., Dr. med.
Klinikum Steglitz, Freie Universität Berlin
Hindenburgdamm 30, 12203 Berlin, Germany

GORISCH, W., Dr. rer. nat.
Düppelerstrasse 20, 81929 München, Germany

KLAMMERT, R., Dr. med.
Urologische Universitätsklinik, Klinikum Grosshadern
Marchioninistrasse 15, 81377 München, Germany

HOFSTETTER, A. G., Professor Dr. med.
Urologische Universitätsklinik, Klinikum Grosshadern
Marchioninistrasse 15, 81377 München, Germany

KRIEGMAIR, M., Privatdozent Dr. med.
Urologische Universitätsklinik, Klinikum Grosshadern
Marchioninistrasse 15, 81377 München, Germany

LUBOS, W., Dr. med.
Urologische Universitätsklinik, Klinikum Grosshadern
Marchioninistrasse 15, 81377 München, Germany

MÜLLER, G., Professor Dr. rer. nat.
Lasermedizin-Zentrum Berlin
Krahmerstrasse 6–10, 12207 Berlin, Germany

MUSCHTER, R., Privatdozent Dr. med.
Urologische Universitätsklinik, Klinikum Grosshadern
Marchioninistrasse 15, 81377 München, Germany

ROTHENBERGER, K.-H., Dr. med.
Urologische Abteilung, Klinikum Landshut
Robert-Koch-Strasse 1, 84034 Landshut, Germany

SCHMELLER, N., Professor Dr. med.
Urologische Universitätsklinik, Klinikum Grosshadern
Marchioninistrasse 15, 81377 München, Germany

SCHNEEDE, P., Dr. med.
Urologische Universitätsklinik, Klinikum Grosshadern
Marchioninistrasse 15, 81377 München, Germany

WAIDELICH, W., Professor Dr. rer. nat.
Becker-Gundahl-Strasse 32, 81479 München, Germany

WONDRAZEK, F., Dr. rer. nat.
Fachhochschule München
Lothstrasse 34, 80335 München, Germany

Theoretical Principles

Theoretical Principles

1 Laser Physics

W. WAIDELICH

The laser is a unique source of energy whose potential can only be imagined. Comparable to the initial use of electricity a century ago, the laser has brought significant changes in many areas, especially medicine and industry. Unlike electricity, however, the laser has no counterpart in nature – it is purely an invention of the human mind. Whereas Roentgen immediately recognized the medical potential of X-rays, this was not the case for the first laser emissions, whose medical applications had to be discovered.

1.1
Historical Development of the Laser

In 1917 Albert Einstein predicted that under certain conditions a light wave in a quantum mechanical system could be amplified through the process of stimulated emission.

Ordinary light waves rapidly diffuse and become less intense as they propagate. A normal spherical wavefront traveling through space is attenuated with the square of the distance traveled, while a wavefront passing through a nontransparent medium is attenuated by absorption and scattering. These facts led earlier researchers to conclude that the amplification of light waves was not a practical goal.

In 1960 Theodore Maiman used a ruby crystal to achieve the light amplification that was theoretically predicted more than 40 years earlier. Figure 1.1 shows the basic components of this first functional laser. When a cylindrical ruby rod with plane-parallel end surfaces was irradiated by a high-intensity flashlamp, the light amplification process was initiated in the perpendicular direction.

The beam emanating from the device was monochromatic, nondivergent, and coherent. The term "maser," referring to microwave amplification, was already in use at the time, so Maiman's light amplifier was called a "laser"–an acronym that expresses both the function of the device and its underlying principle: *light amplification by the stimulated emission of radiation.*

To date, thousands of materials have been investigated for use as potential lasing media. Many different laser systems have been developed and tested. Here we consider only the few systems that have found medical applications.

Fig. 1.1. Experimental setup for the first functional laser. A ruby crystal rod with plane-parallel ends is pumped with energy from a flashlamp to induce stimulated emission from the rod

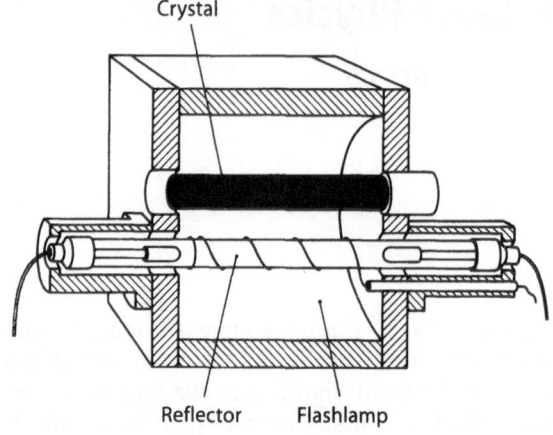

Crystal

Reflector   Flashlamp

To help in understanding the generation of laser light and its unique properties, the basic physical principles of lasers are reviewed below.

1.2
Physical Principles

1.2.1
The Wave-Particle Duality

Light spans a limited range of frequencies between radio waves and x-rays in the broad electromagnetic spectrum. The physical description of light may draw upon the wave model or the particle (corpuscular) model, depending on the type of phenomenon under study (wave-particle duality). The wave model is useful for mathematical descriptions of the propagation and superimposition of waves (diffraction and interference). The particle model is useful for explaining the interactions of light with matter, especially the generation of light (photon emission), absorption, and scattering.

A *wave* is a periodic, temporally and spatially oscillating process characterized by a wavelength λ and a frequency ν. The propagation velocity c of a wave is given by:

$$c = \lambda \nu \tag{1}$$

For electromagnetic waves traveling in a vacuum (or in air), the propagation velocity is $c = 3 \times 10^8$ m/s.

In the *particle model*, light is regarded as a stream of quantum particles called photons. The quantum energy of a photon is defined by:

$$E_{photon} = h\nu \tag{2}$$

where ν is the frequency of the light, and h is a universal constant called Planck's constant, equal to 6.6257×10^{-34} Js (joule-seconds).

1.2.2
Spontaneous Emission

The absorption and emission of light are described in terms of the classic Bohr model of electron orbitals and the particle nature of light. When the energy level of an orbital electron is changed by the amount ΔE, a quantum of light, or photon, of energy $h\nu$ is either absorbed or emitted. The law of energy conservation leads to the equation:

$$\Delta E = h\nu \tag{3}$$

Of the many electrons orbiting an atomic nucleus, only the outermost electron participates in photon interactions. Normally, unless energy is added from an external source, this electron is in a low-energy resting state called the ground state, E_0 (Fig. 1.2a). The *absorption* of a photon raises the electron from the ground state E_0 to a higher energy level, E_1 (Fig. 1.2b). The photon is exterminated, and its energy is converted to the excitation energy of the electron:

$$h\nu S E_1 - E_0 \tag{4}$$

The *emission* of a photon occurs when a previously excited electron releases energy and reverts to the lower-energy ground state (Fig. 1.2c). The electron returns *spontaneously*, without interacting with a radiation field, to its ground state within a period of 10^{-8} s. In the process it emits a photon whose quantum energy equals the difference in energy between the two energy states of the electron:

$$E_1 - E_0 = h\nu \tag{4'}$$

The energy released from the electron, $\Delta E = E_1 - E_0$, determines the quantum energy hn of the emitted photon, so it also determines the frequency n and, according to Eq. 1, the wavelength λ of the light that is produced.

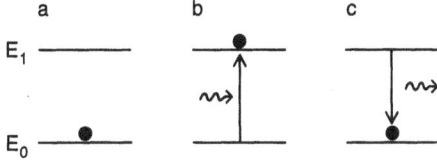

Fig. 1.2a–c. Energy states of an orbital electron during interaction with a photon: **a** ground state of the electron, **b** absorption of a photon, **c** emission of a photon. *Points*, Electrons; *wavy arrows*, photons

1.2.3
Stimulated Emission

Einstein postulated the phenomenon of stimulated emission in which one incoming photon is amplified to two outgoing photons through atomic collisions. For stimulated emission to occur, an excess percentage of atoms must be excited to a higher energy state (population inversion). The return of the electrons to the lower ground state in this situation does not occur randomly (spontaneously) but is stimulated by emissions from neighboring atoms. A spontaneous photon emission (Fig. 1.3a) provides the initial impetus for the subsequent cascade of stimulated emissions (Fig. 1.3b–d).

The population inversion necessary for stimulated emission cannot be achieved in the simple two-level scheme described above (Figs. 1.2, 1.3). An equal distribution of atoms between the two states is all that can occur in a bilevel system. Stimulated emission and absorption would cancel out, and the medium would be transparent. At least one more energy level must be added (Fig. 1.4) to produce an excess of atoms that can occupy an excited energy state for the relatively long period of 1 ms. This "metastable level" provides the necessary reservoir for excited state atoms.

As Fig. 1.4 shows, the addition of energy by the absorption of photons of quantum energy $h\nu = E_2 - E_0$ briefly raises the electrons from the ground state to the highest excited state, E_2. From there the electrons "fall" within 10^{-8} s to the metastable level, E_1, which serves as the reservoir for stimulated emission; the electrons do not emit radiation as they enter this level. Laser radiation having the quantum energy $h\nu = E_1 - E_0$ is produced by the stimulated decay of the electrons from the metastable level to the ground state.

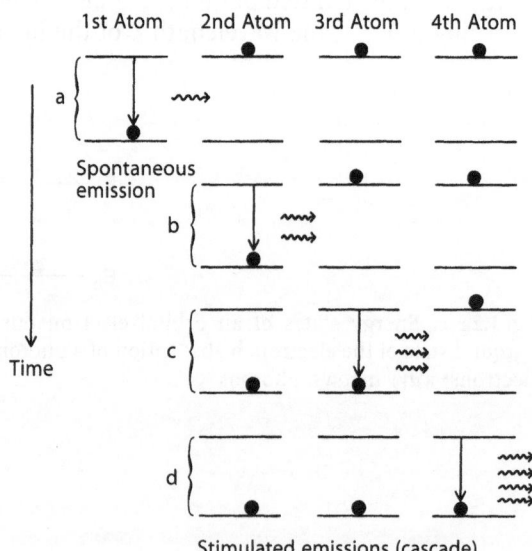

Fig. 1.3a–d. Stimulated emission (cascade), shown for four excited atoms. **a** Spontaneous emission. **b–d** Secondary emissions stimulated by the initial spontaneous emission

Fig. 1.4. Energy states in a three-level laser

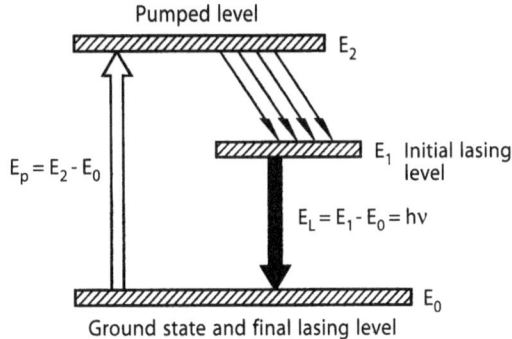

Fig. 1.5. Energy states in a four-level laser

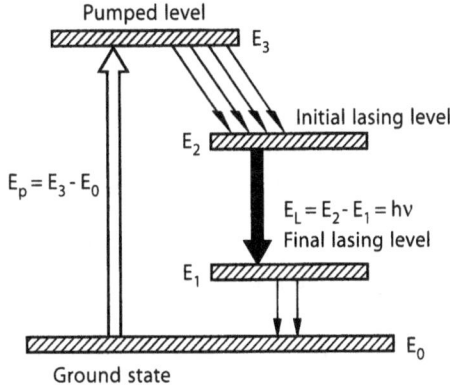

The three-level model shown in Fig. 1.4 formed the basis of the original ruby laser. Special cases aside (semiconductor lasers, excimer laser), the operation of all other lasers is based on at least four different levels of electron energy. The model of a four-level system is shown in Fig. 1.5. Since the lower level E_1 is vacant, only a few electrons must occupy the upper level E_2 for a population inversion to occur. This minimizes the power output necessary to induce stimulated emission.

Conditions are far less favorable in the three-level laser, where inversion must be induced against a ground state that is fully occupied. Maiman's pioneering achievement is all the more impressive when we consider that he was able to generate the first laser beam despite the extremely unfavorable trilevel energy system in a ruby rob. Since its discovery in 1960 the ruby laser has retained its unique status as the only functioning trilevel-energy laser that has ever been developed.

1.3
The Physical Components of a Laser System

A laser consists of three basic components: the lasing medium (active medium), the pump source, and the resonator. The lasing medium and

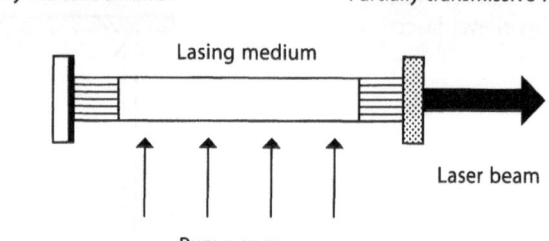

Fig. 1.6. Basic components of a laser

resonator mirrors together form the laser resonator (optical resonator), into which energy is pumped from a suitable energy source. Figure 1.6 shows the basic design elements of a laser system.

1.3.1
Lasing Medium

In principle, light amplification by stimulated emission can occur in all aggregate states of matter (solid, liquid, gas). Accordingly, lasers can be classified as follows:

- Solid-state lasers (crystals, glasses)
- Semiconductor lasers
- Dye lasers (dyes in liquid solution)
- Gas lasers

As an exception, a *free-electron laser*, a laser beam of any desired wavelength can be generated without an active medium by alternately changing the direction of an electron beam. It would exceed our scope to delve further into this complex laser design.

1.3.2
Pump Source

The lasing medium may be pumped with optical or electrical energy to induce a population inversion.

Optical Pumping

In optical pumping, the laser is pumped with light energy that, when absorbed, raises the atoms from their ground state to a higher energy state.

The first ruby laser developed by Maiman was pumped with noncoherent light from a gas-discharge source (flashlamp). This generates laser pulses that are synchronous with the flash pump. A solid-state laser can be operated in the continuous-wave (CW) mode by pumping it with continuous light from an arc lamp. Because only the range of wavelengths corresponding to the energy characteristics of the active medium is utilized to produce laser light, significant portions of the broad-band emission of a gas-discharge lamp are lost going into heat. Adequate cooling is needed to keep the laser at a constant operating temperature. Semiconductor diodes whose emission is spectrally matched to the absorption of the lasing medium minimize this waste heat generation by unutilized pump energy. Very compact laser systems can be designed according to this principle, although semiconductor diodes significantly limit the power that can be generated.

Electrical Pumping

Gas lasers can be pumped with high-frequency electromagnetic radiation or with a high-voltage gas discharge triggered by a direct current.

A very simple type of electric pump is employed in semiconductor lasers. Excitation is produced directly by an electric current. The conduction of current through laser diodes operated in the forward direction causes a population inversion of charge carriers at the pn junction after a certain current density is reached. Recombination of the charge carriers (negative electrons and positive holes) leads to the emission of a coherent laser beam. Semiconductor lasers are extremely small, as indicated by the millimeter-scale dimensions shown in Fig. 1.7.

1.3.3
Optical Resonator and Laser Oscillator

The process of stimulated emission is increased by enclosing the active medium between two mirrors so that the stimulated emissions are reflected back and forth in the axial direction (Fig. 1.6). In its simplest form, an opti-

Fig. 1.7.
Semiconductor laser

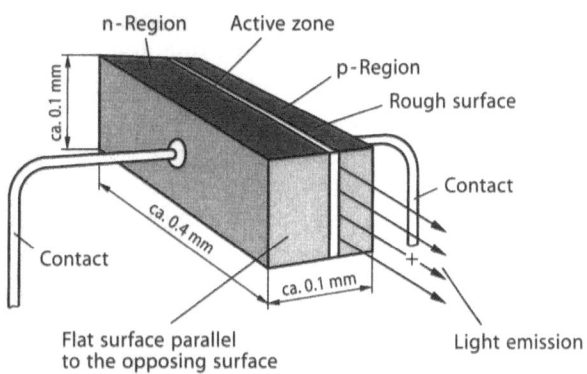

cal resonator consists of two plane-parallel mirrors, one of which is completely reflective while the other is approximately 2 % transmissive to allow the laser light to escape.

Laser Oscillator

Photons traveling through the optical resonator collide with atoms in the lasing medium, stimulating the emission of more photons that have the same energy, direction, and oscillation as the incident photon. When the pump output exceeds a threshold value, the laser becomes self-exciting. The lasing medium and optical resonator together constitute the laser oscillator.

The cascading photons in the lasing medium create an amplification effect that is limited by the number of atoms in the excited state. Standing waves are set up between the resonator mirrors, and undamped, intrinsic modes of oscillation occur within a self-exciting oscillator.

Axial Modes of the Resonator

The distance L between the mirrors in the resonator cavity is a whole multiple of one-half the wavelength of the standing waves (Fig. 1.8):

$$L = n \, \lambda/2 \quad n = 1, 2, 3... \tag{5}$$

This equation can be combined with Eq. 1 to give the resonant frequency of the nth order:

$$v_\eta = n \, c/s \, L \tag{6}$$

The frequency difference between two adjacent modes of oscillation, given by the equation:

$$\Delta v = c/2 \, L \tag{7}$$

depends on the length L of the resonator but does not depend on the frequency itself. The vertical lines in Fig. 1.9 mark the location of the axial modes. The center frequency n_0 is determined by the frequency of the laser transmission. Since, for various reasons, the laser transmission has a finite spectral bandwidth, all axial modes below the amplification profile, but above the loss line v can become operative.

Fig. 1.8. Standing waves between two resonator mirrors

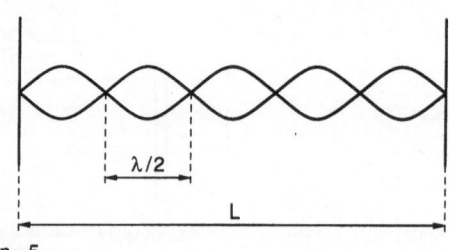

$n = 5$

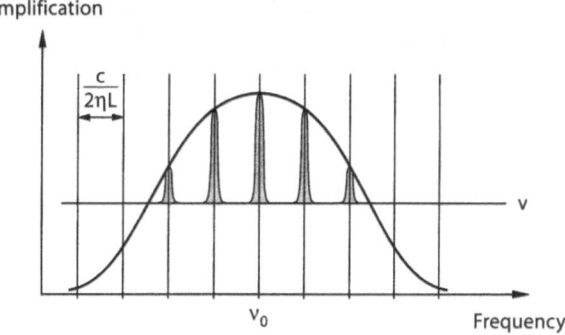

Amplification

$$\frac{c}{2\eta L}$$

v_0

Frequency

Fig. 1.9. Axial modes of a laser oscillator. The vertical lines indicate the possible axial modes. In reality, the modes drawn into the graph are the only ones that are excited

Transverse Electromagnetic Modes (Intensity Profile of the Laser Beam)

An electromagnetic wave is composed of two mutually perpendicular oscillations of the electric and magnetic field. The transverse electromagnetic mode (TEM) of a laser beam characterizes the intensity profile of the beam by designating the extinction points of the standing waves that are perpendicular to the laser axis. A spatially resolving radiation detector mounted perpendicular to the path of the laser beam (e.g., photographic film) can document the TEM structure of the beam. Various transverse modes are illustrated in Fig. 1.10.

The uniformly exposed spot at upper left represents the fundamental mode (uniphase mode), designated TEM_{00}. The ideal mode of operation of a surgical laser is the fundamental TEM_{00} mode, as this yields a beam with a compact, circular cross section. However, even slight contamination of a

Fig. 1.10. Transverse electromagnetic modes

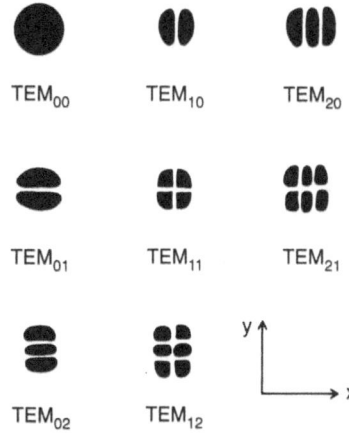

TEM_{00} TEM_{10} TEM_{20}

TEM_{01} TEM_{11} TEM_{21}

TEM_{02} TEM_{12}

resonator mirror can alter the modal structure, producing a TEM_{10} mode or higher order modes. This means that the laser beam is split into two or more components and is no longer homogeneous.

1.4
Units and Exposure Parameters

The most important operational parameters of a laser are the power P, expressed in watts (W), and the amount of energy E that is delivered in time t (E=P×t). Energy is measured in joules (J). The effect at the impact site is defined in terms of the power density or energy density that is delivered to the site per unit area (in cm^2). In medical parlance, these quantities are commonly referred to respectively as "intensity" and "dose" (Table 1.1).

A proper distinction is not always drawn between "power" and "energy." Power describes the ability to deliver energy, while energy is the product of power and time. A laser operating at a power of 1 W for 1 s has an energy output of 1 W×1 s= 1 Ws= 1 J. An exposure time of 20 s would deliver 20 J of energy. Conversely, a laser source delivering 1 J of energy in 1 s would have a power output of 1 J/s= 1 Ws/s= 1 W.

If the source can deliver 1 J of energy in less than 1 s, its power would be greater than 1 W. For example, if a laser emits 1 J in 1×10^{-3} s, its power would be 1×10^3 W= 1 kW. The shorter the time in which a given amount of energy is emitted, the higher the power. Thus, a laser delivering 1 J of energy in 10^{-9} s would have a power output of 10^9 W= 1 GW.

Table 1.1. Physical units of laser radiation

Term	Symbol	Unit
Power	P	W (watts)
Time	t	s (second)
Energy	E=P×t	J (joule) 1 J= 1 Ws
Area	F	cm^2
Power density (intensity[a])	I=P/F	W/cm^2
Energy density (dose[a])	B=E/F	J/cm^2

[a] Term commonly used in medicine.

1.5
Generating Short Pulses of High Intensity

1.5.1
Q-Switching

The power output of a laser can be significantly increased by Q-switching (where Q is the quality factor of the optical resonator). As the laser is pumped, energy emission from the resonator is suppressed until a high level of population inversion is reached. A relatively low pump rate increases the percentage of atoms occupying the metastable level, so when stimulated emission finally occurs, the laser emits a short energy burst of very high intensity ("giant pulse"). The timing of resonator function is controlled by rotating mirrors or by electrooptical or photochemical switches.

In normal operation, a ruby laser emitting 1 J of energy in a pulse of 1 ms duration has a power output of 1×10^3 W. The same laser operating in the Q-switched mode can generate pulses of 10 ns duration at 1×10^8 W.

1.5.2
Mode Locking

A mode-locked laser can emit even shorter pulses in the picosecond range, producing an extremely high power output measured in gigawatts. This is achieved through synchronization or "locking" of the various axial modes in the resonator cavity. Mode locking can be produced in the resonator by a modulation cell that is ultrasonically controlled at a frequency of c/2L (where c is the velocity of light and L is the resonator length). This acoustoontic modulator functions as a time-varying diffraction grid that causes periodic damping of the laser emission. Intermittent suspension of the damping at intervals of 2 L/c generates a corresponding sequence of short laser pulses.

1.6
Properties of Laser Light

Laser light has several unique properties that distinguish it from conventional light sources such as incandescent bulbs and gas-discharge lamps:

- Coherence
- Monochromaticity
- Small divergence
- High power density

1.6.1
Coherence and Monochromaticity

Conventional light sources operate by the disordered, spontaneous emission of energy from individual atoms. Short, damped wave trains emanate from the atoms. All the emissions are independent of one another, and the light is noncoherent.

By contrast, the laser emits a narrow beam of *coherent light* consisting of undamped sine waves that are perfectly in phase. Coherence determines the interference properties of waves. To understand coherence and the distinc-

Fig. 1.11a–e. Wavefronts of noncoherent light from an incandescent bulb and of coherent laser light.
a–d Incandescent bulb.
a Noncoherent light from a thermal emitter.
b Pinhole aperture to enhance spatial coherence.
c Spectral filter to enhance temporal coherence. **d** Enhanced spatial and temporal coherence.
e coherent Laser beam

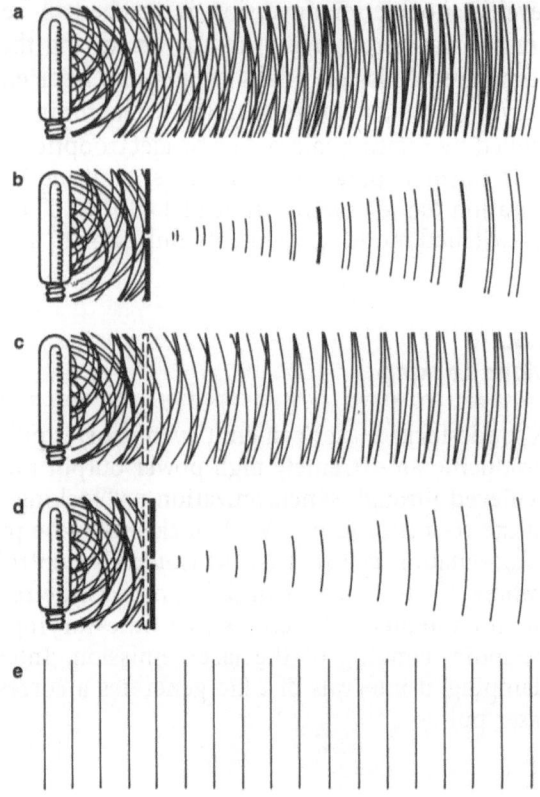

tion between spatial and temporal coherence, Fig. 1.11 illustrates how noncoherent light from an ordinary light source can be made partially coherent. At the top of Fig. 1.11a, a thermal light source is emitting light at various wavelengths in a statistically diverse mix of phases. The *spatial coherence* of the light can be enhanced by passing the beam through a pinhole aperture (Fig. 1.11b). Its *temporal coherence* is improved by passing it through a narrow-band spectral filter (Fig. 1.11c). When both measures (the pinhole and filter) are combined, they theoretically produce a coherent wave train (Fig. 1.11d), but this is achieved at the cost of an almost total attenuation of the power output, which tends toward zero. Only a laser (Fig. 1.11e) can deliver a coherent wave train of high power.

The *monochromatic* nature of laser light is shown in Fig. 1.12, which compares normal fluorescent light (ordinary light) with laser light. The graph shows the optical properties of a ruby crystal, the active medium used in the first laser. Colorless aluminum oxide comprises the matrix of the ruby, which derives its red color from the presence of chromium ions. When these Cr^{3+} ions are excited by optical energy, they respond with the well-known phenomenon of fluorescence, yielding a broad band of emis-

Fig. 1.12. Light emission from a ruby: ordinary broad-band fluorescent light compared with the discrete, monochromatic emission of a laser

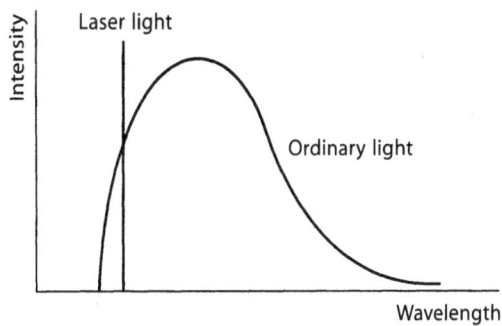

sions over a large range of wavelengths. By contrast, the laser emits light over a very narrow band of wavelengths, i.e., the light is highly monochromatic.

1.6.2
Beam Divergence

Lasers emit a narrow, almost parallel beam that, due to physical laws, is slightly divergent as a result of diffraction. The shorter the wavelength of the radiation and the larger the beam diameter at the exit mirror, the less the beam diverges. The divergence angle of diffraction-limited laser beams ranges from 5×10^{-4} cGy (He-Ne gas laser) to 0.5 cGy (semiconductor laser).

1.6.3
Beam Diameter and Power Density

The beam diameter is defined by an imaginary circular cross section that encompasses 86 % of the laser power. In the ideal case of a gaussian distribution (Fig. 1.13), the diameter is defined as the value at which the field

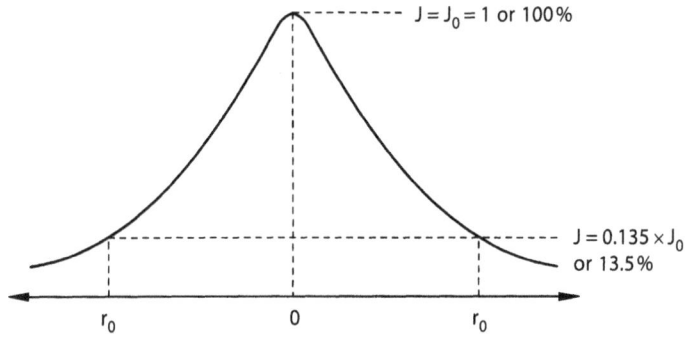

Fig. 1.13. A gaussian bell curve describes the ideal intensity distribution of a laser operating in the TEM_{00} mode

Alfons G. Hofstetter (Ed.)
Lasers in Urological Surgery

1.8
Operational Parameters of Laser Systems

1.8.1
Temporal Parameters

Lasers can operate in the continuous-wave mode (CW, known also as the continuous-beam mode) or in the pulsed mode.

1.8.2
Spectral Parameters

Fixed-frequency lasers selectively emit at a single wavelength or at multiple concomitant wavelengths based on the energy level of the lasing medium. (The argon laser, for example, can operate strictly on one line or on all lines simultaneously.)

Tunable lasers can be tuned to any desired frequency within a specified range.

With dye lasers that emit over a broad spectral band, a narrow range of wavelengths can be selected by placing a prism within the laser resonator. Only light that is reflected along the axis of the resonator cavity is amplified by stimulated emission (Fig. 1.14). The laser can be tuned to the desired amplified wavelength by rotating the prism.

Another way to tune laser light is by changing the temperature of lasing media whose energy states are temperature-dependent. This can be performed with semiconductor lasers, for example.

Passing light through certain crystals (e.g., lithium niobate) can double the frequency of the laser emission through nonlinear effects (*frequency doubling*). This can transform the invisible IR emission of the Nd:YAG laser ($\lambda = 1064\,\text{nm}$) into visible green light ($\lambda = 532\,\text{nm}$).

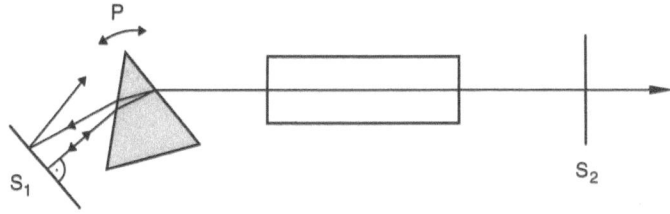

Fig. 1.14. The light from a dye laser can be tuned with a rotating prism. *P*, Prism; S_1, S_2, mirrors

1.8.3
Delivery Systems for the Application of Laser Energy

With few exceptions, a delivery system is needed for a comfortable handling of the laser beam between the generator and the target site. Laser light in the spectral range from UV (200 nm) to the visible and near-infrared regions (2500 nm) can be delivered through flexible fiberoptic waveguides. Outside this region and especially in the mid-infrared range, the beam must be transmitted with the aid of articulating mirrors (see Fig. 1.15).

The universal use of lasers in medicine, including endoscopic applications, was made possible by the development of thin, flexible delivery systems. The physical principle of light transmission through fibers made of quartz glass or other materials is based on a total internal reflection with no lateral escape of light. The light rays are reflected at the interface of the fiber with the surrounding medium (cladding) and continue to propagate through the fiber until they escape at the end. To transmit light in this way, the fiber must have a higher refractive index than the cladding or coating material.

The laser beam that emanates from the end of the fiber shows a relatively high degree of divergence. This problem can be minimized by focusing the beam and by maintaining a short standoff distance from the target. The problem of divergence can be avoided altogether by using a *contact tip* on the distal end of the optical fiber for the direct contact cutting of tissue. Advances in delivery systems have been a critical factor in the development of new laser applications in medicine. Fiber tips with special emission characteristics have become available for specialized forms of laser treatment.

Ongoing and future laser research aims at miniaturizing laser systems to sizes far below 1 cm^3, which will allow the laser to be integrated directly into surgical and analytical instruments (Schmitt 1995).

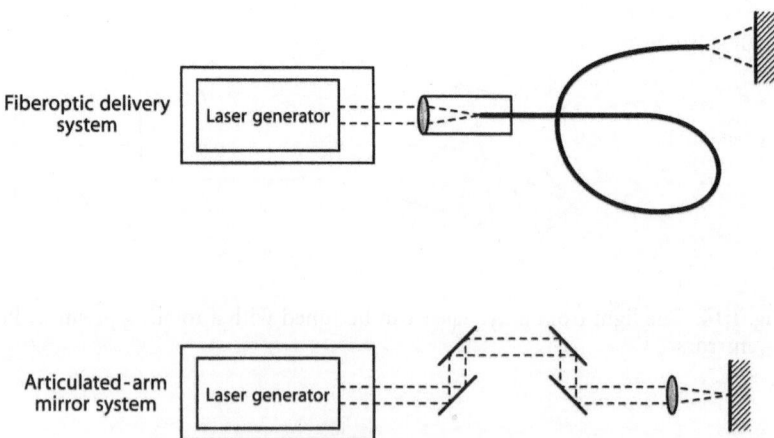

Fig. 1.15. Laser delivery systems: flexible fibers and articulating mirrors

1.9
Interaction of Laser Energy with Biological Tissue

1.9.1
Physical Principles

Mechanisms of Energy Transfer

There are several processes by which laser energy can interact with biological systems:

1. Ionization by high-energy photons or by multiphoton processes. Effects: chemical reactions, luminescence, heat
2. Electron excitation by UV and visible radiation. Effects: chemical reactions, luminescence, heat
3. Induction of oscillation and rotational modes by IR radiation. Effect: heat

When IR radiation is applied to tissue (process 3), all the energy is transformed into heat. With electronic excitation (processes 2 and 3), only a portion of the energy is converted to heat. Heat production results from an increase in the kinetic energy of the tissue molecules.

Laser-Tissue Interactions

The interactions of the laser beam with biological tissues depend on the wavelength-dependent optical properties of the lased tissue. The primary determinant of the laser action is the absorption coefficient of the tissue, for only radiation that is absorbed produces an effect. The relaxation coefficient and scattering coefficient are additional factors that determine the absorption and penetration of laser energy.

The complex structure of biological tissues makes it difficult to offer a precise description of the propagation of laser light. However, we can give an approximate description based on the simplified model of a thin tissue layer.

Laser light striking a tissue layer can undergo any of four physical processes:

- *Reflection* of the light at interfaces between media with different refractive indexes
- *Scattering* by molecules, particles, organelles, and cells
- *Absorption* by molecules, cells, and chromophores
- *Transmission* of the remaining energy

The attenuation of a laser beam that has the intensity J_0 as it enters the tissue depends on the thickness of the tissue layer:

$$J = J_0 \times e^{-Kd} \tag{8}$$

where $K = \alpha + \beta$.

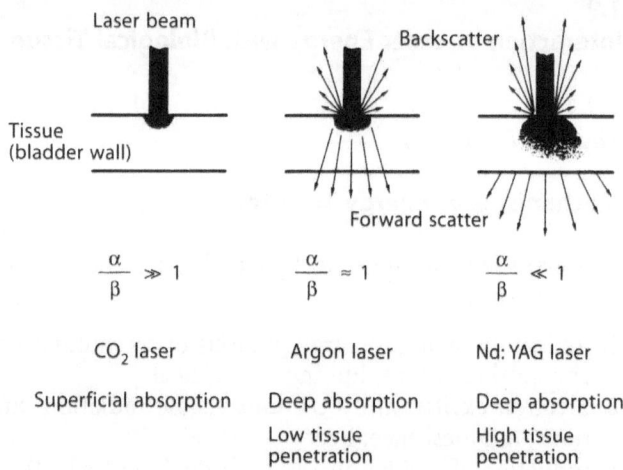

Fig. 1.16. Wavelength-dependent laser beam attenuation in tissue due to absorption α and scattering β (Hofstetter and Frank). CO_2 laser energy is strongly absorbed, while Nd-YAG laser energy is strongly scattered. Argon laser energy undergoes equal scattering and absorption

The extinction coefficient K represents the sum of the absorption coefficient α and the scattering coefficient β.

The reciprocal of the extinction coefficient has length as its dimension. For $d = 1/K$, the intensity falls to $1/e = 38\%$, the value for the "mean penetration depth."

Given the wavelength dependence of the absorption and scattering coefficients, different types of laser energy produce different tissue effects, as shown in Fig. 1.16. Absorption is predominant with the CO_2 laser, scattering with the Nd:YAG laser.

Since tissue is composed mainly of water, the absorption coefficient of water is critical for laser applications based on thermal effects. Water is transparent in the visible region of the spectrum. Light with a wavelength in the low-infrared region (780 nm) is weakly absorbed by tissue water, but absorption increases substantially past 1400 nm, approaching values on the order of $\alpha = 1000\,\text{cm}^{-1}$. Table 1.3 shows the mean penetration depths in water and blood for three important medical lasers. (The argon laser is use-

Table 1.3. Mean depth of laser penetration in water and blood (with attenuation to $1/e = 38\%$)

Laser	Wavelength (nm)	Water (mm)	Blood (mm)
CO_2	10 600	0.01	0.01
Nd-YAG	1064	100	2.5
Ar	528	10 000	0.03

ful for retinal coagulation owing to its strong absorption by hemoglobin and its very slight absorption by water.)

These lasers have the following specific medical applications based on their absorption and penetration characteristics:

- CO_2: cutting, ablation, vaporization (superficial effect, strong absorption by water and blood)
- Nd:YAG: coagulation, hyperthermia (deep effect, heavy scattering)
- Ar: coagulation (selective absorption by hemoglobin)

These applications can be overlapped by selectively modifying the exposure conditions. For example, the CO_2 beam can be defocused to produce superficial coagulation, while the Nd:YAG beam can be focused for the cutting and ablation of tissue. The holmium:YAG laser ($\lambda = 2120$ nm) is intermediate between the CO_2 and Nd:YAG lasers in its absorption by water. The IR emissions of the Nd:YAG and Ho:YAG lasers can be transmitted down fiber-optic waveguides, making these lasers excellent for endoscopic use. The CO_2 laser is more limited in its applications due to the lack of a (tested) flexible fiber waveguide.

With new lasers that operate at wavelengths between the Nd:YAG and CO_2 lasers, we may be closer to the goal of developing a universal surgical laser that can cut or coagulate when set to different power densities. Besides the holmium laser, the erbium:YAG laser ($\lambda = 2940$ nm) appears to be a promising candidate. Its emission coincides with a strong water absorption band, giving the laser good cutting capabilities. The erbium beam cannot be transmitted through quartz fibers, and for now it appears doubtful that other flexible fiber systems such as As_2S_2 will find practical application.

Table 1.4 shows experimental data comparing the cutting properties of three infrared lasers. The Nd:YAG and Ho:YAG lasers are inferior to the CO_2 laser in their cutting abilities, but they are compatible with flexible fiber-optic delivery systems and thus offer a significantly wider range of applications.

Advanced miniaturized laser systems are small enough to fit into the distal end of endoscopes, overcoming the problem of transmission of the laser beam via fibers. This allows the easy application of the erbium laser beam even in minimally invasive techniques. A further advantage is a very small focus that can increase the power density (Peuser and Schmitt 1995).

Table 1.4. Depth of cut obtained with infrared laser scalpels

Laser	Nd:YAG	Ho:YAG	CO_2
Wavelength	1064 nm	2120 nm	10 600 nm
Transmission through 0.1 mm of H_2O	90 %	50 %	0.1 %
Depth of cut (at 25 W, 1.5 mm/s)	0.2 mm	0.5 mm	3.5 mm

1.9.2
Mechanisms of Biological Effects

The bioeffects of surgical lasers may be thermal or nonthermal.

Thermal Effects

Photocoagulation

The temperature rise in the tissue depends on the duration of exposure to the laser energy and the thermal properties of the tissue, i.e., its specific heat capacity, heat conduction, and convection (flowing blood).

When the laser energy is applied in a short pulse, heat is not dissipated from the impact site, and negligible cooling occurs. The large temperature gradient between the laser spot and its surroundings gives rise to mechanical stresses that cause ablation with no heating of the surrounding tissue.

When the energy is applied over a longer period, the heat spreads to surrounding tissues in a spherical pattern. The thermal pulse (laser application) is long compared with the thermal relaxation time (time needed to establish an equilibrium between heat input and removal).

These two boundary cases demonstrate the different ways in which the peak temperature can decline with distance from the center of the laser spot. A quantitative analysis shows that the temperature rise caused by a short laser burst is a function of energy ($\Delta T \sim E$) while that caused by a more prolonged application is a function of power ($\Delta T \sim P$), i.e., the rate at which energy is delivered to the system.

When a critical temperature T_c is reached, irreversible tissue damage occurs. The duration of the temperature pulse is determined either by the length of the heating pulse or by the diffusion time for cooling of the irradiated tissue. In the case of hemoglobin, for example, T_c varies no more than 10 °C when the pulse width varies over 11 orders of magnitude.

Irreversible tissue damage does not occur below about 45 °C. As the temperature rises to 45°–50 °C, there is damage to enzymes and the cell membrane accompanied by edema formation.

When tissue heating is continued for several seconds, the coagulation of cell protein occurs when the temperature reaches 60 °C. Protein denaturation is visibly manifested by a whitish discoloration of the tissue. This temperature is sufficient to cause capillary sealing, so hemostasis is also obtained. The Nd:YAG laser beam is excellent for coagulation owing to its deep penetration. Interstitial laser coagulation represents a relatively new application of this principle.

Photothermal Cutting and Vaporization

At $T = 100\,°C$ the strong absorption of infrared radiation by water leads to boiling of the tissue water, cell rupture and dehydration, and tissue shrinkage. Continuing the exposure past the boiling point of the cell water does not cause a further rise in temperature initially, because the applied energy is consumed as evaporative heat in changing the material from the liquid to the vapor phase. Once all the water has been vaporized, the temperature starts to climb again. Beyond about $150\,°C$ carbonization occurs, and increased energy absorption by the charred surface promotes a relatively sharp rise in temperature. Temperatures higher than $400\,°C$ are associated with vaporization, burning, and excavation.

The heavy absorption of the CO_2 beam by water creates a potent thermal effect that is excellent for incising tissues that contain water. However, since the beam cannot be transmitted via fiberoptics, the CO_2 laser is limited to line-of-sight applications in which the beam can be manipulated with mirrors. Only Nd:YAG and Ho:YAG lasers are universally suitable for endoscopic applications.

Nonthermal Effects

Photoablation. In this process tissue is ablated by the disruption of molecular bridges ("cold vaporization"). The applied energy is utilized to break chemical bonds and vaporize the fragments. Because there is no heat transfer to surrounding tissues, it is possible to make extremely precise tissue incisions without heating. The photons in the laser light must have sufficient quantum energy to disrupt chemical bonds. Therefore photoablation is performed with UV-emitting excimer lasers, which generate pulses of extremely high power density (GW/cm^2).

Photodisruption. When the power density is raised to extremely high levels, "optical breakdown" occurs as a laser-induced plasma rapidly forms, expands, and collapses. The mechanical shock waves induced by this explosive process are useful for the fragmentation of urinary stones. Dye lasers and alexandrite lasers are effective for photodisruption. The advanced state of this technology is illustrated by systems that can discriminate stones from other tissue based on an analysis of the backscattered light. Full-power lithotripsy pulses are fired only when low-level backscatter has identified the target as a stone.

Photochemical Effects. Prolonged exposure to laser light of low power density can induce chemical reactions between chromophoric compounds without heating the tissue. In addition to endogenous chromophores, photosensitizing compounds can be administered and selectively retained in certain cells for laser diagnosis and treatment.

These processes form the basis for photodynamic diagnosis and therapy. Hematoporphyrin derivatives have been widely studied for use as photosensitizing agents in diagnostic and therapeutic oncology. The violet beam of the nitrogen laser ($\lambda = 406$ nm) is used diagnostically to excite a red fluorescence in these compounds, and the red light from a dye laser or gold vapor laser ($\lambda = 628$ nm) is used for tumor treatment. Experimental research is currently being carried out on other tumor-specific photosensitizers (e.c. δ-amino-levolinic acid).

Laser Biostimulation. Laser light of low power density is successfully used in many cases for the biostimulation of wound healing and the treatment of pain. There are also reports of immunological effects and applications in stimulation therapy and acupuncture. Particularly good results have been reported with red light from the He-Ne laser and infrared light from the Ga-As semiconductor laser. Although many studies have been conducted, more information is needed before we can understand the nature of the biostimulatory response in man. Above all, it is unclear whether lasers operated at low power settings are a useful but nonessential energy source for this type of therapy. Since coherence appears to be unimportant, the only advantage of laser light is its monochromaticity. However, it is very costly to generate monochromatic light free of unwanted spectral components, especially thermal radiation, from a noncoherent light source. Since there is still no proof that biostimulatory effects are laser-specific, there is an obvious benefit to using cost-effective laser systems (especially laser diodes) for nonthermal phototherapy.

References

Anders A, Altheide HJ (1989) Laser. Thieme, Stuttgart

Barnes FS (1971) Biological damage resulting from thermal pulses. In: Laser applications in medicine and biology. Plenum, New York London

Beesley MJ (1976) Lasers and their applications. Taylor & Francis, London

Dändliker R (1971) Laser. Aargauer Tagblatt, Aarau

Dinstl K, Fischer PL (1981) Der Laser. Springer, Berlin Heidelberg New York

Frank F (1992) Biophysical fundamentals of laser applications in medicine. In: Bastert G, Wallwiener D (eds) Lasers in gynecology. Springer, Berlin Heidelberg New York

Gurs K (1970) Laser. Umschau, Frankfurt am Main

Haina D, Waidelich W (1976) Kohärente Optik. Berichte Physikalisches Institut, TH Darmstadt

Hofstetter AG (1988) Laserkoagulationsbehandlung von Urotheltumoren im oberen Harntrakt. In: Schaller J, Hofstetter A (eds) Endourologie. Thieme, Stuttgart

Hofstetter AG (1988) Laserkoagulationstherapie des Harnblasenkarzinoms. In: Schüller J, Hofstetter AG (eds) Endourologie. Thieme, Stuttgart

Hofstetter AG, Frank F (1979) Der Neodym-YAG-Laser in der Urologie. Roche, Basel

Karamanolis S (1990) Das ABC der Lasertechnik. Elektra, Munich

Martelluci S, Chester AN (1984) Laser photobiology and photomedicine. Plenum, New York

Parrish JA (1980) Photomedicine potentials for lasers. In: Pratesi R, Sacchi CA (eds) Photomedicine and photobiology. Springer, Berlin Heidelberg New York

Peuser P, Schmitt NF (199R) Diodengepumpte Festkörperlaser. Springer, Berlin Heidelberg New York
Rother C (1993) Dornier-Medizintechnik. Personal communication
Schmitt NF (1995) Abstimmbare Mikrokristall-Laser. Shaker, Aachen
Sutter E, Schreiber P, Ott G (1989) Handbuch Laserstrahlenschutz. Springer, Berlin Heidelberg New York
Waidelich W (1972) Kohärente Optik. Strahlenschutz in Forschung und Praxis, vol XII. Thieme, Stuttgart
Wolbarsht ML (1971) Laser applications in medicine and biology. Plenum, New York

2 Safety Aspects of Laser Surgery

F. Frank and F. Wondrazek

2.1
Hazards Posed by Laser Systems

The medical applications of laser systems are constantly expanding. Medical laser systems currently in use consist of the laser base unit, a delivery system, and application instruments whose design depends on the particular indication. The medical-surgical utilization of lasers requires the implementation of appropriate safety precautions to protect the patient, physician, and support personnel from laser injuries. The goal of clinical laser therapy is the denaturation of organic tissue using a laser beam that develops sufficient intensity to produce the desired effect within the treatment area. However, measures must be taken to ensure that laser emissions outside the treatment area are so attenuated in their intensity that they pose no hazard to the laser operator and other personnel. This includes adequate safeguards against any inadvertent beam impacts that may occur outside the operative field.

When all necessary safety precautions are followed, lasers can be used safely in medical settings without jeopardizing the patient, physician, or personnel.

2.1.1
Electrical Hazard

Since the laser base unit has an electric power supply, electrical safety is an issue. When a laser system has been manufactured in accordance with proper technical standards and is operated in compliance with established standards of practice, the electrical hazard is no greater than that posed by any conventional, electrically powered medical equipment.

2.1.2
Biological Hazards

Lasers emit a concentrated beam of electromagnetic energy that poses a laser-specific hazard to biological media. While the beam parameters of wavelength, power, energy, and pulse width are critical to the success of a procedure, they also determine the degree of hazard to the eyes and skin of the laser operator, patient, and support personnel.

The eye is particularly vulnerable, since the ocular lens can focus laser light to a highly concentrated spot on the retina. Hence, laser safety is primarily a matter of eye protection (Hillenkamp et al. 1980; Sliney and Wolbarsht 1981; Winburn 1985; Sliney and Trokel 1993).

Wavelength

Laser wavelengths below 380 nm in the ultraviolet (UV) range of the spectrum are strongly absorbed by biological tissue, posing a hazard to the cornea and lens of the eye as well as exposed skin. All the UV wavelengths, as with ionizing radiation, exert a cumulative biological effect. The ultraviolet region is subdivided into UV-A, UV-B, and UV-C:

- UV-A laser light, occupying the range from 315 to 389 nm, penetrates several millimeters into the skin and causes weak pigmentation. When this light impinges on the eye, most is absorbed by the lens and leads to cataract formation.
- UV-B, ranging from 280 to 315 nm, causes erythema and secondary pigmentation of the skin. Ocular exposure causes photokeratitis.
- UV-C, in the range below 280 nm, can penetrate only a thin superficial tissue layer. Its effects are similar to those of UV-B.

UV radiation can also produce cellular effects leading to late sequelae. UV light promotes premature aging of the skin due to the degeneration of cutaneous cells, and it predisposes to various forms of skin cancer.

The visible region of the spectrum occupies the range from 380 to 780 nm. Wavelengths above 380 nm are absorbed by the anterior media of the eye, and the retina is insensitive to wavelengths shorter than 780 nm. Visible laser light poses an extreme hazard to the retina due to the focusing action of the eye. The power density of incident rays increases from the cornea to the retina in proportion to the ratio of the area of the pupil to the area of the retinal image. All light passing through the pupillary aperture, which ranges from 5 mm to at most 7 mm in size, is projected onto the retinal surface. The diameter of this projected image is determined by the refractive limit of the pupil; 10 μm would be a typical value for the nondivergent rays of a laser beam. Thus, as the beam passes from the cornea to the retina, its power density is amplified by a factor of 5×10^5. The bioeffects of laser light in the short-wave region of the spectrum are determined chiefly by photochemical processes, whereas effects in the long-wave region are determined by the thermal activity of radiation absorbed by the tissue.

The injurious effects of infrared (IR) radiation, occupying the range between the visible and microwave regions, are entirely thermal in nature. IR radiation, as with UV, can be subdivided into three ranges based on its absorption by tissue.

Lasers operating in the IR-A range of 780–1400 nm are especially hazardous to the eye, because these wavelengths can penetrate to the retina without producing a visual impression of light.

Light in the IR-B range of 1400–3000 nm is so strongly absorbed by water in the anterior segment of the eye that it cannot reach the retina. However, it can induce cataract formation when absorbed by the lens and iris.

IR-C wavelengths above 3000 nm are very strongly absorbed by water and are stopped well short of 1 mm penetration (Fig. 2.1).

The potential injurious effects of laser light on the various structures of the eye are wavelength-dependent based on differences in the absorption characteristics of the cornea, lens, chambers, and retina (Holzinger et al. 1978; Fig. 2.2).

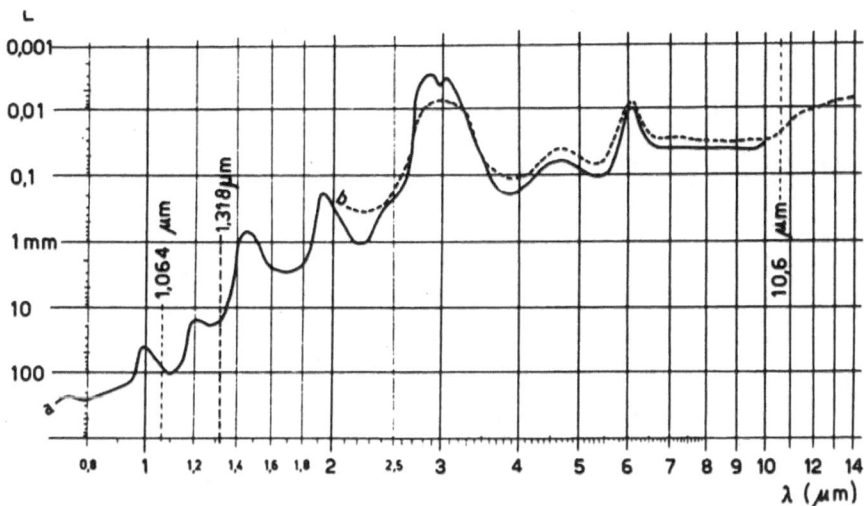

Fig. 2.1. Depth of penetration of electromagnetic radiation of various wavelengths in water. (*a* From Bayly et al. 1963; *b* from Bramson 1968)

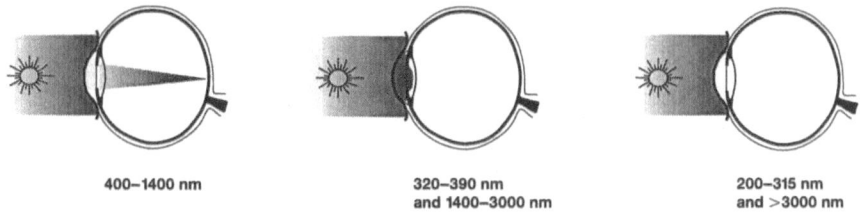

Fig. 2.2. Potential for laser injury to various structures of the human eye

Exposure Time

The exposure time and pulse duration are important variables in determining the physical and biochemical effects of laser irradiation. Exposure to a continuous-wave laser beam for a period significantly longer than the thermal relaxation constant of the tissue causes a temperature rise that is proportional to the delivered power. Through heat conduction, an equilibrium is established between the delivery and dissipation of energy. The critical parameter in this case is the beam intensity, measured as power per unit surface area (power density). If the biological time constants are greater than the exposure time, the effect is proportional to the dose, and the critical parameter is the energy per unit surface area (energy density). As the duration of the laser pulse is shortened, other mechanisms of tissue injury can come into play. For example, the thermal expansion caused by a rapid temperature rise can trigger the formation of acoustic shock waves. Vaporization processes are another mechanism that can induce shock waves. As the pulse duration is reduced further, the electric field strength becomes so intense that an electrical avalanche breakdown can occur in tissue. This breakdown results from the massive acceleration of free electrons that are present in the tissue and, at high electric field intensities, are generated by multiphoton processes. The various tissue-disrupting mechanisms are dependent on the intensity and duration of the exposure (Sutter et al. 1989; Fig. 2.3).

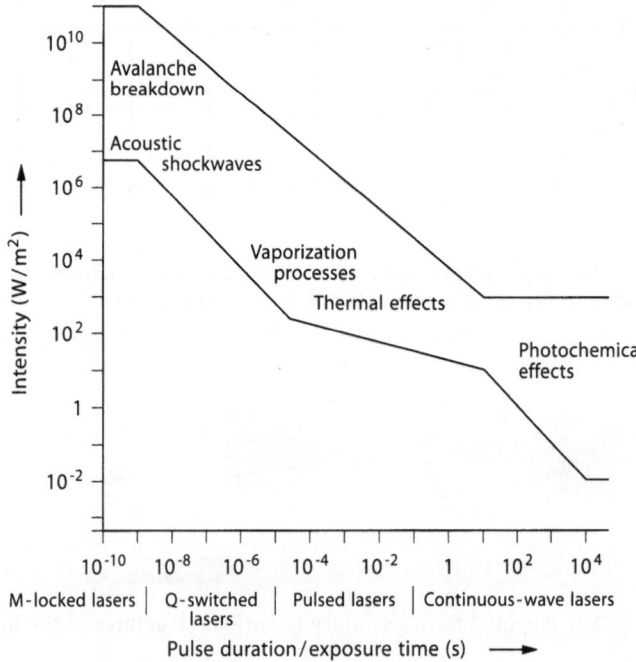

Fig. 2.3. Dependence of various mechanisms of laser injury on the duration and intensity of exposure

Characteristics of the Radiation Source

Besides physical beam parameters such as wavelength, pulse duration, and power, the size and distance of the radiation source also affect the degree of hazard. The least favorable situation is one in which a direct or reflected laser beam is considered to originate from a point source. This produces the smallest possible spot on the retina, depending on the resolving power of the eye. A far more favorable situation is one in which the source is relatively large in area and exceeds the resolution limit of the eye. For equal power densities impinging on the cornea, the beam intensity at the retina is always higher from a point source than from a more expansive source.

We must also consider hazards that can result from the reflection of laser light from medical instruments and other surfaces. Specular reflections are extremely hazardous, because they duplicate the point-source characteristics of the laser beam. Diffuse reflections, however, distribute the laser light over a large spatial angle and make it appear to originate from a more extended source.

2.1.3
Chemical Hazards

Besides direct impacts, laser can produce secondary effects that are hazardous to patients and personnel. A therapeutic laser has sufficient intensity to ignite flammable materials. Combustible materials that are used in the operative area (e.g., solvents, ventilation gases, draping materials) may ignite or explode when struck by a laser beam. Breakdown products generated during laser treatment can also jeopardize the health of patients and personnel (Allgemeine Unfallversicherungsanstalt 1984).

2.2
Technical Standards and Classification

A classification of laser systems has been devised, along with a set of technical standards and limits, to make it easier for users to follow proper safety precautions and thus ensure the safer use of laser equipment.

2.2.1
Exposure Limits

Experimental studies on the thresholds of injury to the eye and skin have made it possible to establish limits for permissible exposure. These limits, called MPE (maximum permissible exposure) values, show a complex dependence on wavelength and exposure time. This complexity is illustrated by graphs in which the maximum permissible exposure levels for the eye (Fig. 2.4) and skin (Fig. 2.5) from point sources of various wavelengths are plotted against time. The safe limits for the skin and eye in the visible and near-IR spectral regions differ from one another mainly in the amplification effect caused by the focusing action of the ocular lens. This action

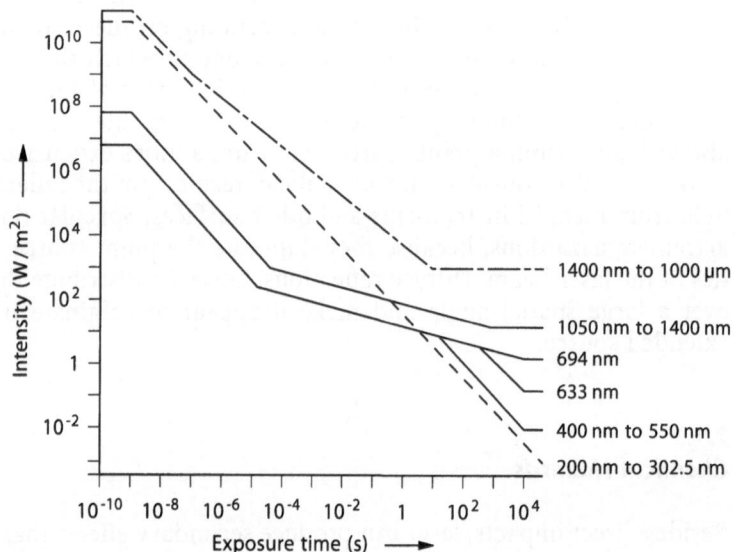

Fig. 2.4. Maximum permissible exposure levels for the eye as a function of exposure time

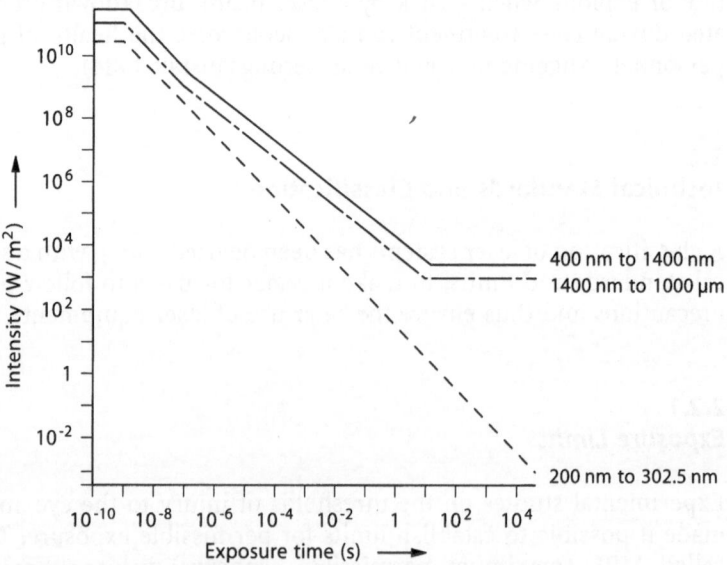

Fig. 2.5. Maximum permissible exposure levels for the skin as a function of exposure time

does not occur at UV and far-IR wavelengths, so the limits are equal. The exposure limits are twice as high for visible and near-IR light as for the far-IR region, because far-IR beams have very high penetration, and a significant portion of the energy is backscattered and escapes from the tissue. This results in a lower specific volume absorption for a given intensity, leading to higher permissible exposure limits.

2.2.2
Laser Area

The laser area (controlled laser area, control area) refers to the enclosed space in which there is a potential for exceeding the maximum permissible exposure during normal laser use. The extent and boundaries of the laser area can be accurately determined only by the measurement of radiation exposure levels.

The medical-surgical applications of lasers range from superficial, external treatments and laser use in open surgery to endoscopic and interstitial laser treatments in organs and body cavities. These varied applications are associated with highly diverse configurations of the nominal laser area.

When special application systems such as endoscopes are used, the laser area is confined to the interior of the patient's body. When freehand instruments and handpieces are used, the laser area may encompass the entire operating suite (Frank and Halldorsson 1982).

2.2.3
Technical Standards

Technical standards are the foundation for practical laser safety. The basic technical standards for laser safety are contained in Publication 825-I of the International Electrotechnical Commission, "Safety of laser products: equipment classification, requirements and user's guide" (IEC 1993).

This document is identical to the 1994 publication DIN EN 60825–1 from the German Standards Institute on the "Safety of laser equipment," which introduces a four-class system for categorizing laser hazards. A major section deals with standards for the manufacturers of laser equipment. Another main section presents guidelines for users of laser equipment. Built-in safety filters and protective eyewear are covered in publication DIN EN 207 (1993), "Personal eye protection." Electrical safety is covered in the German Electrical Engineers (VDE) publication DIN 57836/VDE 0836 (1977), "VDE standards for the electrical safety of lasers and laser systems." These technical standards provided the basis for establishing codes and specifications for safe laser use. For personnel safety, the new Accident Prevention Code on "Laser emissions" has been in force since April 1988. It deals with the generation, transmission, and application of laser energy and presents very detailed guidelines for users. Patient safety is addressed in the

1985 Medical Equipment Code, which specifies the responsibilities of the operator and the manufacturer.

Laser safety standards published by the American National Standards Institute (ANSI) are similar in content to IEC publication 825-I. The standards in ANSI publication Z136.1, "Safe Use of Lasers" (ANSI 1980), correspond to the IEC 825 document. The recommendations in Z136.3 deal with the "Safe use of lasers in the health care environment" (ANSI 1988).

2.2.4
Laser Classes

As noted above, the 1994 publication DIN EN 60825-1 defines classes of lasers based on physical parameters such as power output, wavelength, and mode of operation (continuous or pulsed). The class of a laser characterizes the degree of hazard associated with its use, with higher numbers signifying a greater degree of hazard. Each laser class is associated with a specified range of possible exposures.

Class 1 lasers have a very low power output and are intrinsically safe, meaning that there are no circumstances in which exposure could exceed maximum safe limits. Class 1 CW lasers emitting at 400–550 nm should have a power output no higher than 0.39 µW. Special safety measures are not required for class 1 lasers. Enclosed lasers of a higher class are also placed in this category, although personnel who manipulate the laser enclosure are at risk for exposure to higher emissions.

Class 2 lasers are low-power units with a visible beam that may be pulsed or continuous. The power output or energy output of these lasers is limited to class 1 levels for exposure times up to 0.25 s. The power limit is 1 mW for lasers operating in the continuous-wave mode. The only eye protection needed for class 2 lasers is the natural aversion response with reflex closure of the eyelids.

Class 3a lasers have a power output limited to 5 mW for visible light at wavelengths of 400–700 nm. Directable laser systems and systems that are repeatedly pulsed in the same spectral range may emit at five times the class 2 levels, but the power density of the visible beam may not exceed 25 W/m^2 at any location. This means that, with a pupil diameter of 7 mm, no more than 1 mW of power would enter the eye from a continuous-wave source. Wavelengths outside the range of 400–700 nm may be up to five times the class 1 power limit, but the power density may not exceed the maximum permissible exposure for the eye. When optical aids such as telescopes are used, class 3a lasers are hazardous to the eye regardless of their emission spectra. When optical aids are not used, reflex closure of the eyelids affords adequate eye protection from laser light at visible wavelengths.

With class 3b lasers, a direct beam impact to the eye is always hazardous. It is safe to view diffuse reflections from unfocused pulsed lasers, and diffuse reflections from continuous-wave lasers are safe when viewed from an adequate distance. Visible or invisible continuous-wave lasers may not exceed a power output of 0.5 W, and pulsed lasers must have an energy output less than 10^5 J/m^2. Lasers at the upper limit of class 3b usually exceed the maximum permissible exposure values for the skin. They pose a fire hazard when used in the presence of highly flammable materials.

Class 4 lasers are high-power units whose power outputs exceed the limits for class 3b. Even diffuse reflections from these lasers are hazardous to the eye and skin. They can cause skin injury and pose a significant fire hazard.

2.3
Safety Measures

Most medical lasers are class 3b or class 4 devices. To ensure safety, a variety of safety measures must be implemented at the manufacturing, organizational, and operational levels (Allgemeine Unfallversicherungsanstalt 1985; Laser Institute of America 1983; Ringelhan et al. 1988).

2.3.1
Equipment Safety

Every medical laser must come equipped with certain safety features. These include a key-operated switch and a connection for a safety door interlock. The unit should produce an audible and/or visible warning signal when the beam is activated. There should be a built-in system for measuring the energy dose delivered to the patient with an accuracy of ±20 %, and there should be a warning signal to indicate improper dosing. The point of laser impact on the tissue should be indicated, usually by means of a coaxial, low-wattage aiming beam.

2.3.2
Organizational Measures

In every hospital that uses lasers, a laser safety officer should be appointed who is fully responsible for all safety measures. Only specially trained personnel should be allowed to work with laser equipment. All persons who are involved in the operation of a laser must be educated about the effects of laser radiation, its hazards, and necessary protective measures. The operational safety of the laser should be checked before the unit is activated, and a laser log should be kept. Equipment maintenance should be performed as directed, and regular safety inspections should be conducted. Startup of the laser system and any laser accidents should be reported to the hospital administration and to authorities concerned with worker safety.

Fig. 2.6. Laser warning sign

2.3.3
Installation

The laser area in medical laser applications covers the entire space in which maximum permissible exposure levels may be exceeded due to direct laser impacts, reflections from instrument surfaces, or incidents such as the careless handling or breakage of fiberoptic components. Often the laser area encompasses the whole operating suite, but it can be reduced by setting up curtains or partitions as barriers. Warning signs should be posted at entryways to the controlled laser area (Fig. 2.6). Door interlocks should trigger an automatic laser shutdown if unauthorized personnel enter the controlled area. To prevent unauthorized laser use, the key should be removed from the key switch and stored in a safe place.

2.3.4
Eye Protection

All persons present in the controlled laser area must wear protective eyewear that completely shields the eye from potentially hazardous rays. The optical density of the filter material should be sufficient to attenuate the laser beam well below the maximum safe levels for corneal exposure. As specified in the DIN publication on "Personal eye protection," the filter and frame must be able to withstand laser irradiation for at least 10 s (DIN EN 207, 1993). The protective eyewear should transmit as much visible light as possible and should cause minimal color distortion. Laser goggles should be comfortable to wear, provide a large field of vision, and fit snugly against the face.

Any optical instruments used in conjunction with the laser, such as endoscopes or microscopes, must be equipped with protective eye filters if the light may exceed maximum permissible levels.

To avoid hazardous reflections, medical instruments used in the laser area should have a matte black finish and should have curved outer surfaces of low radius. Flat surfaces should be avoided. The surface roughness needed to produce a diffuse reflection depends on the laser emission spectrum. Walls and floors in the laser area should not have highly polished surfaces, and appropriate window coverings should be installed.

2.3.5
Protection from Chemical Hazards

Given the risk of fire and explosion associated with the use of high-power lasers, flammable liquids should not be used during laser procedures. Precautions against fire and explosion hazard should be taken whenever lasers are used in proximity to organs, body cavities, or hoses that may contain combustible fumes or gases. Hoses that carry oxygen or flammable anesthesia gases should be made of laser-proof material or sheathed with material that is resistant to laser impact. Auxiliary equipment and draping materials that may be inadvertently exposed to laser emissions during surgery must be flame-retardant. Towel drapes can be dampened to reduce the risk of being ignited by the laser beam.

Laser smoke should be evacuated as close to its site of origin as possible, as it may cause adverse health effects and hamper visibility.

2.3.6
Patient Protection

Damage to the patient's eyes and skin from inadvertent beam impact outside the operative field can be prevented by covering the endangered areas. When a laser beam with high tissue penetration is used, underlying organs, nerves, and blood vessels should be protected from accidental injury by carefully controlling the power output and the duration of the exposure.

2.4
Summary

When used properly, medical lasers and accessory equipment are no more hazardous than any other electrically powered medical devices. Because of laser-specific hazards to the eyes and skin, maximum permissible exposure levels have been defined and serve as a basis for establishing appropriate safety measures.

The potential laser hazard varies with power, energy, and wavelength, so lasers are assigned to different classes that have specific safety implications. Class 1 lasers are intrinsically safe, meaning that it is not hazardous to look directly at the laser light. With class 2 lasers, reflex closure of the eyelids protects against irreversible injury. With class 3a lasers, the beam may damage the eye when viewed through optical instruments; with class 3b, only a diffusely reflected beam can be viewed with safety. A class 4 laser beam is hazardous to eyes and skin even when reflected diffusely.

Most laser systems in medicine are class 4 lasers, and some are class 3b. Safety measures include organizational precautions, protective eyewear, and protective eye filters when optical instruments are used.

References

Allgemeine Unfallversicherungsanstalt (1984) Experimentelle Studien zur Sicherheit bei der Anwendung des Lasers in der Medizin. Schriftenreihe, vol 1/84. Vienna

Allgemeine Unfallversicherungsanstalt (1985) Medizinische Anwendung des Lasers. Merkblatt Ml7, Vienna

American National Standards Institute, ANSI (1980) Safe use of lasers. Standard Z-136.1, New York

American National Standards Institute, ANSI (1988) Safe use of lasers in health care facilities. Standard Z-136.3, New York

Bayly IG, Karth VB, Stevence WH (1963) The absorption spectra of liquid phase H_2O, HDO and D_2O from 0.7 μm to 10 μm. Infrared Physics 3:211–223

Bramson M (1968) Infrared radiation. A handbook for applications. Plenum, New York

DIN 57836/VDE 0836 (1977) VDE-Bestimmung für die elektrische Sicherheit von Lasergeräten und -anlagen. Beuth, Berlin

DIN EN 207 (1993) Persönlicher Augenschutz. Beuth, Berlin

DIN EN 60825-1 (VDE 0837) (1994) Sicherheit von Laser-Einrichtungen. Beuth, Berlin

Frank F, Halldorsson T (1982) Untersuchungen zur Sicherheit bei der klinischen Anwendung des Neodym-YAG-Lasers. Biomed 4:30

Hillenkamp F, Pratesi R, Sacchi CA (1980) Lasers in biology and medicine. Plenum, New York

Holzinger G, Kroy W, Schreiber P, Sutter E (1978) Schutz vor Laserstrahlen. Schriftenreihe Arbeitsschutz, no 14, Bundesanstalt für Arbeitsschutz und Unfallforschung, Dortmund

IEC (1993) Safety of laser products: Equipment classification, requirements and user's guide, publication 825-1. Bureau Central de la Commission Electrotechnique Internationale, Geneva

Laser Institute of America (1983) Lasers safety guide. Toledo

Medizingeräteverordnung (1985) Verordnung über die Sicherheit medizinisch-technischer Geräte. Bibliomed, Melsungen

Ringelhan H, Senz RG, Berlien HP, Müller G (1988) Laser sicher angewandt. Krankenhaus Techn, vol 24

Sliney D, Trokel S (1993) Medical lasers and their safe use. Springer, Berlin Heidelberg New York

Sliney D, Wolbarsht M (1981) Safety with lasers and other optical sources. Plenum, New York

Sutter E, Schreiber P, Ott G (1989) Handbuch Laser-Strahlenschutz. Springer, Berlin Heidelberg New York

Unfallverhütungsvorschrift (1988) Laserstrahlen VBG 93. Heymanns, Cologne

Winburn DC (1985) Practical laser safety. Dekker, New York

3 User Certification, Equipment Safety, and Laser Safety Officer*

B. Fuchs, H.-P. Berlien, G. Müller, and W. Gorisch

3.1
Certification Program of the German Society for Laser Medicine

Since the laser was first introduced into medical diagnosis and treatment, there has been a virtual explosion of new technology in this field. Not only are lasers an effective new addition to the therapeutic armamentarium, they are also a cost-effective modality that can help to hold down the burgeoning costs of health care.

However, as with any sophisticated new technology, there are problems in qualifying the personnel who must work with the technology and become proficient in its use.

The medical applications of lasers fall into three broad categories:

- Use of the laser as a primary therapeutic modality, as in photodynamic therapy or laser angioplasty
- Use of the laser as an optional auxiliary instrument, such as the laser-scalpel
- Use of the laser as a diagnostic instrument

In Germany, a set of ordinances called the Medical Equipment Code (MedGV) mandates proper education and training for all users of Group 1 medical equipment, which includes virtually all medical lasers. In addition, document VGB 93 of the Accident Prevention Code on "Laser radiation" requires that each facility using class 4 lasers (the class that includes almost all medical lasers) appoint an expert in laser safety procedures, designated the laser safety officer. Moreover, there is social legislation in Germany that mandates proper qualifications for physicians affiliated with health care funds who provide treatment that requires specialized knowledge and experience.

The medical laser, much as ultrasound, has become a tool that transcends interdisciplinary boundaries. The fact that the laser is used not only in specialty areas but also for interdisciplinary applications (e.g., photodynamic therapy and interstitial thermotherapy) makes it imperative that medical personnel who work with lasers receive comprehensive education and training that goes beyond a single specialty field.

---

* This chapter reviews safety codes, standards, and regulations that apply in Germany.

Recognizing this problem, the German Society for Laser Medicine (DGLM) commissioned a Certification Panel in 1984 whose task was to establish a certification policy. This policy was issued in 1986, corresponding guidelines for a general laser training course were established, and courses were instituted. In 1988 this general training program was approved by the DGLM membership and was expanded by the addition of specialty courses. The European Laser Association (ELA) recommended this type of program, with certain modifications, for the European Community as a whole. At the 1992 meeting of the DGLM, the Society's executive board impaneled a Certification Guidelines Committee to take further steps toward having laser medicine recognized as a subspecialty by the Union of Health Care Fund Physicians and the German Physician's Congress.

The training program officially recommended by the DGLM consists basically of a general course and a specialty course.

The general laser training course is an interdisciplinary course dealing with the basic physical and technical principles of lasers, laser-tissue interactions, basic laser applications, and the principles of medical laser systems and accessory equipment. The course also deals with pitfalls in laser use, legally mandated safety codes and standards, and consequent practical safety measures. The course includes practical exercises with lasers and accessory devices so that participants can observe typical laser effects in tissue specimens.

This course meets the qualification requirements for the laser safety officer and also fulfills the requirements of medical equipment users as specified in the Medical Equipment Code.

The general training phase of the program also serves as a qualifying course for other occupational groups that may assume the duties of a laser safety officer such as medical assistants, hospital technicians, and medical physicists. The training of these personnel at regional centers that specialize in medical laser training is preferred over facilities that also train laser safety personnel for industry, as the latter facilities may not focus on the specific problems of laser use in medicine.

The general phase of the program is followed by a specialized course of training at specialty centers covering such practical issues as indications and contraindications, special application guidelines, and problems in aftercare. The focus of the specialty course is on practical training. In vitro exercises should train participants in the handling of up-to-date equipment that is specific for the specialty area. Emphasis is placed on live video transmissions from the operating room and hands-on training.

Certificates are issued by the DGLM to confirm successful completion of the general and specialty training courses.

3.2
Medical Equipment Code and Laser Safety Officer

W. Gorisch

This section deals with two legal areas that address two fundamentally different areas of responsibility of the attending physician. One involves the *proper therapeutic use* of lasers, the other the *prevention of accidents* to patients and personnel.

The Medical Equipment Code (MedGV) was enacted in Germany on 1 January 1986. The MedGV includes regulations on premarketing inspection and approval by the manufacturer as well as provisions for installation and operation.

Since our focus is on medical lasers, a comprehensive assessment of the MedGV as a whole would exceed our scope, and we shall consider only the MedGV requirements that pertain to laser use.

Section 6, Paragraph 3 of the MedGV states:

Medical devices belonging to Group 1, 3, or 4 shall be used only by individuals who are qualified and proficient in the use of those devices by virtue of their training or their knowledge and practical experience.

Surgical lasers are classified as Group 1 devices, so their use is subject to this requirement. At present, however (November 1993), there is no legal definition of what constitutes adequate knowledge or practical experience on the part of any particular therapist, or the means by which such knowledge and experience are to be acquired.

Because this question actually falls under the heading of the quality and competency of medical services, conflicts would in any case be resolved in a judicial setting. Presumably this would involve assessing all personal efforts that the practitioner has made to gain sufficient expertise and the fund of experience that he or she has acquired and evaluating those qualities in the light of current accepted practice.

To assist in these matters, the German Society for Laser Medicine has established certification guidelines to be used in qualifying medical personnel for laser use [1]. A secondary goal of these guidelines is to promote official recognition of laser medicine as a subspecialty and to provide a basis for establishing guidelines for billing and reimbursement.

The two basic requirements for certification are the acquisition of general proficiency and specialty-oriented proficiency. *General proficiency* is described as covering "the basic physical and technical principles of lasers, laser-tissue interactions, basic laser applications, the principles of medical laser systems and accessories, pitfalls in laser use, legally mandated safety codes and standards, and consequent practical safety measures." *Specialty-oriented proficiency* covers issues such as "indications, contraindications, preparations, and aftercare" relating to laser use, with emphasis on practical exercises and live operating-room demonstrations or transmissions.

There are various institutions in Germany that offer general and specialized laser training and certification for participants (for information, contact the German Society for Laser Medicine, Generalsekretariat Prof. Dr. Landhaler, Dermatologische Klinik der Universität, Franz-Josef-Strauss Alee 11, D-93053 Rebensburg).

The MedGV also requires laser users to follow accident prevention guidelines as stated in Section 6, Paragraph 1:

Lasers shall be installed and operated in strict accordance with the provisions of this Code, generally accepted technological standards, as well as worker-safety and accident prevention codes.

Thus, the MedGV states explicitly that laser users must observe accident prevention codes (actually this is superfluous, given the fact that this requirement is legally mandated elsewhere). This responsibility applies to the hospital administration and all staff involved. Administrators have a particular responsibility to play a lead role in preventing accidents to patients and hospital staff.

The latest version of the "Laser radiation" section VBG 93 of the *Accident Prevention Code* (UVV) is applicable in all settings where lasers are used. A list of the provisions can be obtained free of charge from accident insurance carriers.

The UVV consists of a provisions section and a compliance guidelines section:

The compliance guidelines indicate how the safety goals specified in the Accident Prevention Code can be achieved. They do not rule out equally safe alternative solutions.... The compliance guidelines also include further explanations of provisions contained in the Accident Prevention Code.

Section 6, Paragraph 1 of VGB 93 requires that a laser safety officer be appointed to monitor and enforce specific laser safety measures. The laser safety officer is considered to be technically qualified:

[I]f, based on his specialized training or experience, he has acquired adequate knowledge of the laser or laser system in use and is so thoroughly instructed on the effects of laser radiation, protective measures, and safety provisions that he can evaluate the necessary safety precautions and test their effectiveness. It is recommended that the laser safety officer attend a course for laser safety officers that has been accredited by a professional society or by accident insurance carriers.

Since medical personnel generally have not received special training in laser physics, accident insurance carriers insist that laser safety officers attend an accredited general course. A list of facilities that offer such courses can be obtained from professional societies or insurance carriers.In many cases the hospital administration appoints a responsible physician as the laser safety officer. However, the UVV does not require that a physician or therapist be designated as laser safety officer, nor must the laser user possess the technical expertise of a laser safety officer. For example, a worker from the engineering department or a technically skilled OR attendant may be appointed as the laser safety officer.

A laser safety officer may oversee multiple laser systems, but no more than one laser safety officer should be responsible for a particular laser area.

The specific responsibilities of the laser safety officer depend on the position of the officer within the institution. However, in all cases the laser safety officer must report to the responsible supervisor and hospital administrator with regard to:

- Safety issues involved in the procurement and startup of laser systems
- Support in the determination of safety measures
- Selection of personal protective equipment
- Support in providing necessary technical facilities
- Monitoring compliance with safety measures, especially with respect to the proper use of protective eyewear, barriers, screens, and the posting of area signs
- Informing the responsible supervisor and hospital administrator about equipment problems and defects
- Helping to conduct an annual safety briefing of laser area personnel
- Cooperating with technical personnel for worker safety

If the laser safety officer also holds a supervisory or administrative position, he or she has the additional duties of:

- Establishing technical and organizational safety measures, especially measures that are necessary in the laser area
- Authorizing the performance of equipment service, including temporary shutdown of the laser
- Notifying authorities
- Conducting the safety briefing (at least once a year)
- Instituting appropriate measures in case of accidents

Specific laser safety measures are reviewed in Sect. 2.3.

Reference

Report of the German Society for Laser Medicine (1993) Guidelines for certifying medical personnel for laser use in medicine. Lasermedizin 9:66–71

Clinical Laser Use

4 Thermal Effects of Lasers

4.1
External Genitalia

Lasers are widely used in urology, dermatology, and gynecology for the treatment of various lesions of the external genitalia.

The Nd:YAG laser and the CO_2 laser can both be precisely controlled, and either can be used for cutting or coagulation with favorable postoperative cosmetic results. The laser beam can be transmitted through quartz fibers (Nd:YAG laser) or coupled to a colposcope (CO_2 laser) to treat epithelial lesions of the vagina, rectum, or urethra (Krogh 1990). The laser has emerged as the method of first choice over other modalities, especially in the treatment of HPV-associated cutaneous lesions (e.g., condylomata acuminata; Schneede 1991).

4.1.1
Condylomata Acuminata and Other Viral Skin Lesions

P. SCHNEEDE and A.G. HOFSTETTER

The clinical significance of skin lesions caused by human papillomaviruses (HPV) and their effective laser therapy is based on the fact that human papillomaviruses have been cited as the leading cause of sexually transmitted diseases (European Project 1991; Koutsky et al. 1989; Krogh 1990)and an important precursor of premalignant and malignant disease (Zur Hausen 1987; Wickenden et al. 1985). The selection of a laser system that can provide optimum treatment with a low rate of recurrence is guided by the location and extent of the cutaneous lesions.

Indications

Curative laser treatment is appropriate for:

- HPV-associated skin lesions [condylomata acuminata, Buschke-Löwenstein tumor, flat condylomata, bowenoid lesions, penile (PIN) and cervical (CIN) intraepithelial neoplasia]
- Premalignant lesions and leukoplakia (Bowen's disease, erythroplasia of Queyrat, lichen sclerosus et atrophicus)

Fig. 4.1. a Male urogenital tract. **b** Female urogenital tract

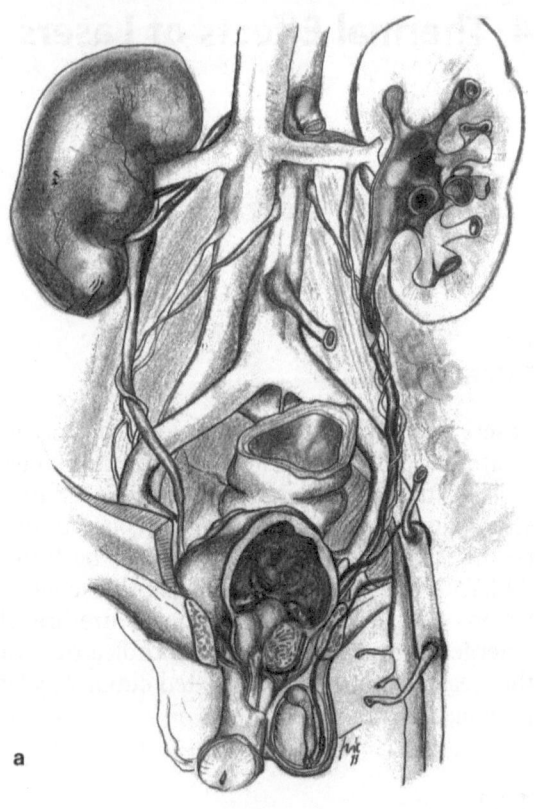

a

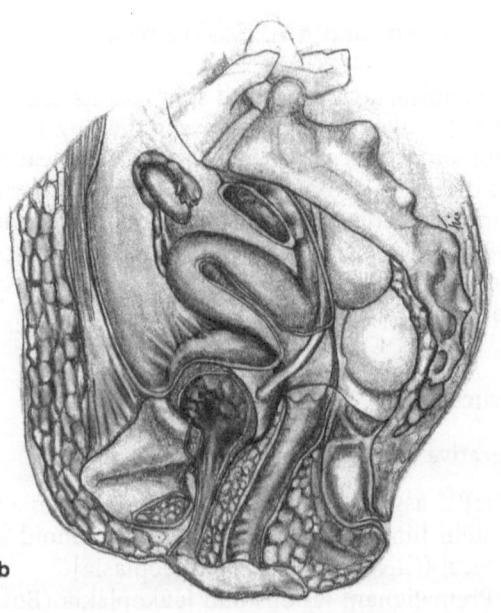

b

- Carcinoma (penile carcinoma, see Sect. 4.1.2)
- Molluscum contagiosum

Preoperative Studies

Flat condylomatous HPV lesions can be demonstrated by applying acetic acid to the external genitalia and inspecting the area under magnification (colposcope, surgical loupe). Other preoperative studies include biopsy and HPV typing, urethroscopy, and the exclusion of infection (fungi, HIV, gonorrhea, *Chlamydia*, *Mycoplasma*, herpes simplex) by culturing or serological testing. Gynecological, proctological, and otolaryngological examinations are also conducted as required

With photodynamic diagnosis (see Sect. 5.2), the instillation of 5-aminolevulinic acid hydrochloride solutions can assist in differentiating penile human papillomavirus lesions from healthy tissue (Fig. 4.2).

Screening for Metastases

Patients with penile carcinoma should be screened for metastatic disease (see Sect. 4.1.2).

Operative Technique

Technical Parameters

- Laser power output: 10–20 W, depending on the size, extent, and location of the skin lesions

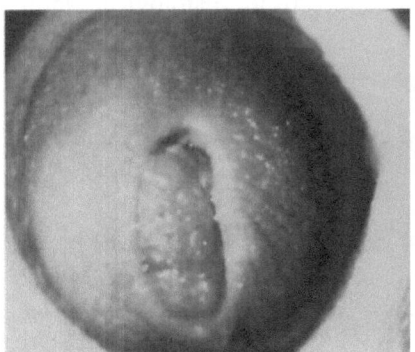 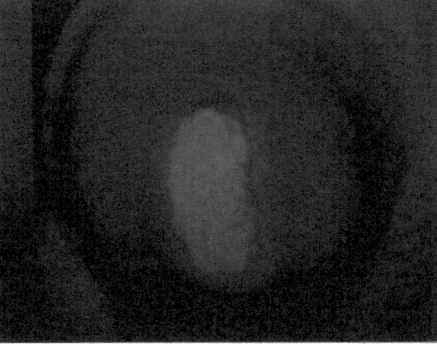

Fig. 4.2. Condylomatum acuminatum of the external urethral meatus before (*left*) and after (*right*) photodynamic diagnosis. The red fluorescence of the HPV lesion sharply demarcates it from healthy adjacent tissue

- Depth of penetration and tissue effects (Fig. 4.2) – Nd:YAG laser:
  - Little superficial absorption
  - Depth of coagulation up to 8 mm; penetration can be controlled by adjusting the power output, exposure time, and surface cooling
- Depth of penetration and tissue effects (Fig. 4.2) – CO_2 laser:
  - High superficial absorption, no coagulation
  - Penetration <1 mm with tissue carbonization and vaporization
- Use on the external genitalia:
  - Nd:YAG laser: used with flexible fiberoptics and a focusing handpiece
  - CO_2 laser: used with an articulated-arm mirror system that directs the beam through a handpiece or colposcope
- Use in the urethra:
  - Only the Nd:YAG laser can be used with water irrigation (CO_2 laser energy is completely absorbed by water and causes vaporization)

Method of Application

- The biophysical properties of the Nd:YAG laser make it better suited for the treatment of exophytic skin lesions (e.g., condylomata acuminata, penile carcinoma; Schneede et al. 1992), while the CO_2 laser or defocused Nd:YAG laser is better for treating lesions at the skin level (e.g., flat condylomatous HPV lesions and premalignant lesions).
- A red helium-neon aiming beam is used with the invisible CO_2 or Nd:YAG laser beam to ensure precision surgery. First the beam is moved around the edges of the skin lesion, then it is swept over the lesion in linear passes until the tissue whitens.
- With extensive preputial involvement, laser treatment should be combined with circumcision.
- For the Nd:YAG laser treatment of exophytic skin lesions (Fig. 4.3):
  - The lesion is lased with a focused beam until it turns pale (Fig. 4.4).
  - The coagulated tissue is removed with a forceps for histological examination (Fig. 4.5a).

Fig. 4.3. Condylomata acuminata involving the urethral meatus and the prepuce

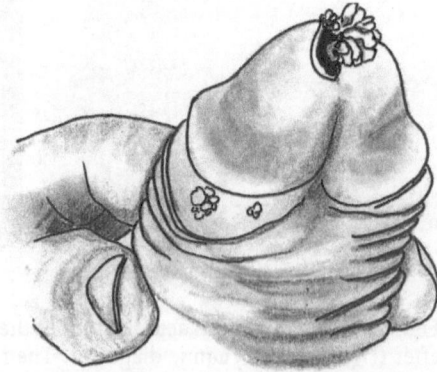

Fig. 4.4. Nd:YAG laser treatment (20 W, defocused) of condylomata acuminata involving the urethral meatus, with evacuation of the laser plume. Appearance following circumcision

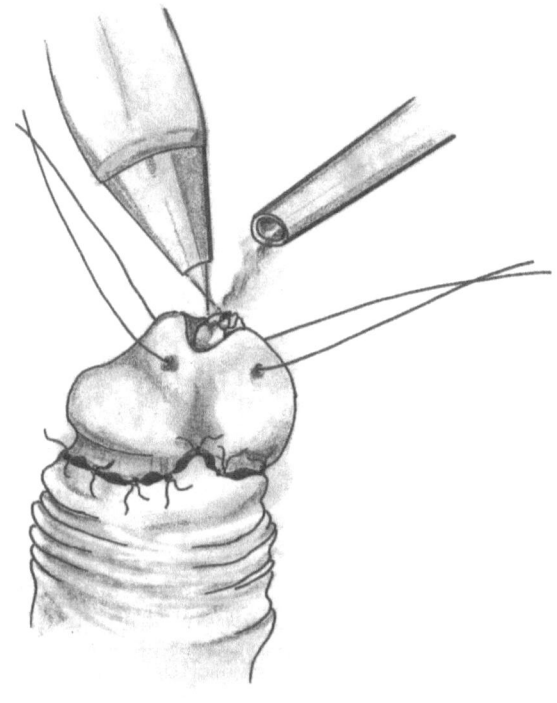

Fig. 4.5. a The coagulated tissue is removed with a forceps. **b** The defocused beam is reapplied to the tumor base

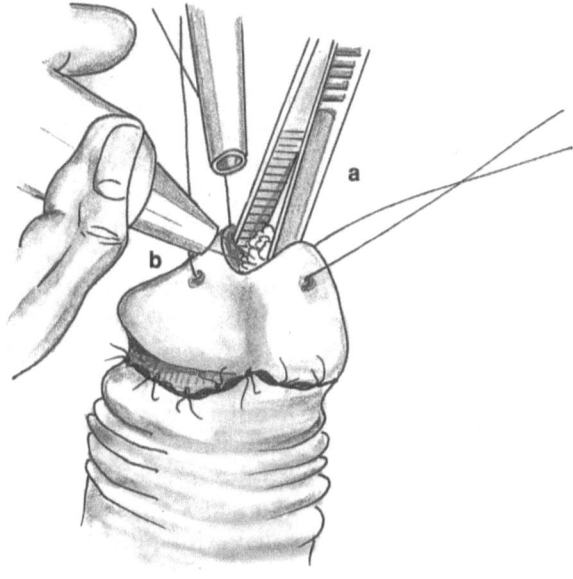

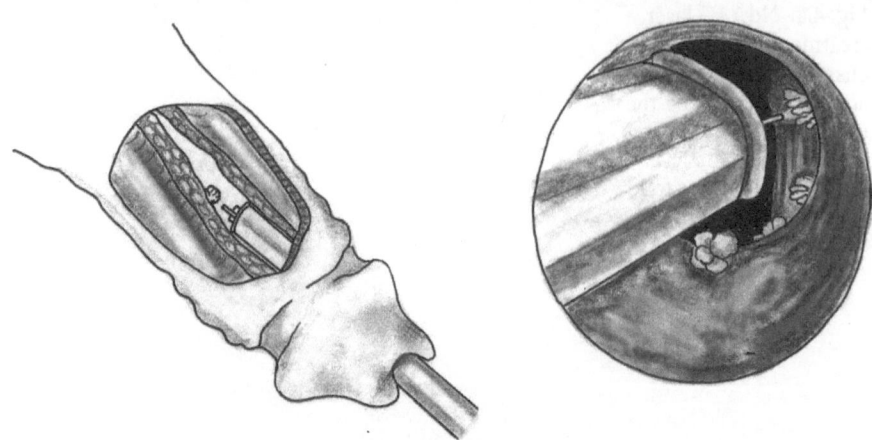

Fig. 4.6. Nd:YAG laser treatment (20 W, focused) of condylomata acuminata involving the urethra

- Finally the base of the tumor is lased superficially with a defocused beam of low power density (Fig. 4.5b).
- For the treatment of flat skin lesions with the CO_2 laser or Nd:YAG laser (10 W, defocused):
  - Flat condylomatous HPV lesions are made visible by applying 5 % acetic acid and waiting for 5 min. The lesions appear as demarcated white areas with punctate vascular markings when viewed under magnification.
  - The CO_2 laser ablation of lesions at the skin level is associated with surface carbonization and a laser smoke plume (Seidl 1992). The plume, which contains viral particles (Garden et al. 1988) and has carcinogenic potential, should be evacuated with a suction line.
  - The Nd:YAG laser should be operated at a low power setting (15–20 W) with a defocused beam (Schneede and Hofstetter).
- Only the Nd:YAG laser is useful for the treatment of intraurethral lesions (Fig. 4.6):
  - The laser beam is applied to the meatus with a focusing handpiece or bare fiber, depending on the location of the urethral condyloma (Fig. 4.7). A forceps or special urethral speculum is used to spread open the meatus in the area of the fossa navicularis (Seidl 1992). Proximal urethral condylomata can be lased through a urethroscope (Fig. 4.8).
  - Lesions that involve the urethra circumferentially should not be treated by circumferential lasing, as this promotes stricture formation. They should be treated with punctate laser impacts. A staged procedure may be required.

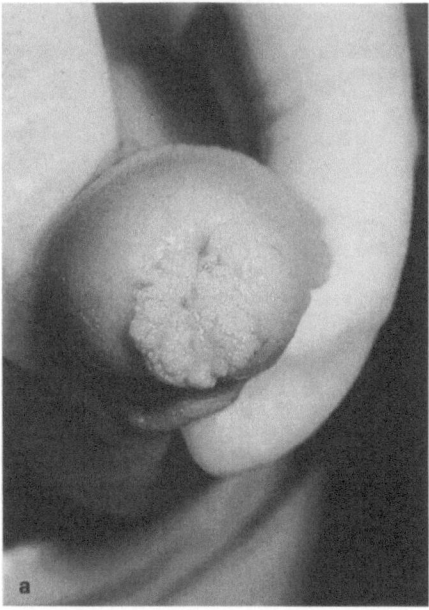

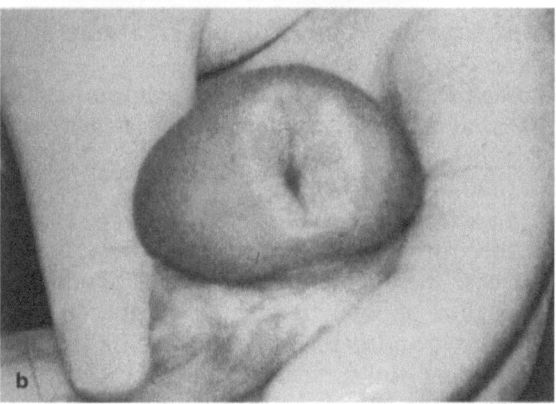

Fig. 4.7. a Solitary exophytic condyloma involving the urethral meatus. **b** Appearance 6 months after Nd:YAG laser treatment (20 W)

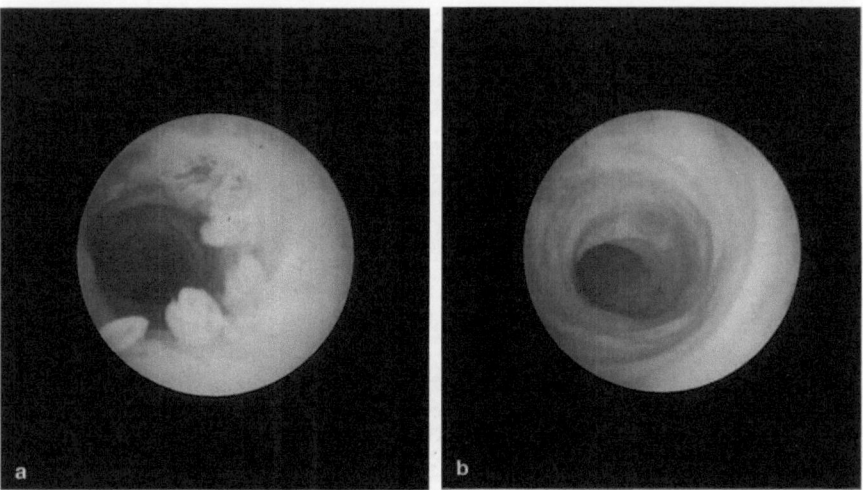

Fig. 4.8. a Intraurethral condylomata acuminata *before* Nd:YAG laser treatment. **b** Appearance 6 months after laser treatment. Only a faint scar is visible

Advantages over Conventional Treatments

- Laser therapy is preferred over conventional methods options owing to its good cosmetic results and low rates of recurrence. Alternative methods include:
  - Cold knife excision
  - Cryosurgery
  - Electrocautery or electrosurgical resection
  - Local therapeutic agents (for HPV infections): 5-fluorouracil, podophyllin, podophyllotoxin, trichloroacetic acid
- Exophytic and flat skin lesions can be treated with equal efficacy while preserving healthy surrounding tissue
- Precise, noncontact laser treatment can be extended to body regions where access is difficult (urethra, vagina, rectum)
- Laser therapy significantly reduces postoperative pain and bleeding

Follow-up

- The wound should be checked after 4–8 weeks, depending on its extent.
- Premalignant and malignant lesions require close follow-up with repeated biopsies and lymph node evaluations.
- The high propensity for recurrence of HPV lesions requires minimum 6-month follow-ups.
- Urethral involvement requires endoscopic follow-up at 4–6 weeks. Postoperative dilatation may be necessary to prevent meatal stenosis.

Contraindications

There are no true contraindications, but the following restrictions should be noted:

- Lesions of the urethra, vagina, or rectum should not be lased circumferentially, and a staged procedure may be required.
- A low power density should be used for the Nd:YAG laser treatment of highly vascularized areas (e.g., the glans penis) or dark pigmented lesions due to the strong energy absorption by these tissues.

Instrumentation (Table 4.1)

- CO_2 laser: articulated-arm mirror system, colposcope, smoke evacuator
- Nd:YAG laser: fiberoptics with focusing handpiece, quartz fibers for use in a urethroscope with a straight-ended sheath
- Instrumentation for photodynamic diagnosis (see Sect. 5.2)

Table 4.1. Laser instrumentation

Laser system	Characteristics
Nd:YAG laser	Technical specifications – Wavelength 1064 nm – Power output: 10–25 W Beam delivery – Through glass fibers in a focusing handpiece or endoscope Tissue effect – Little superficial absorption – Deep penetration with coagulation – Can be used under water
CO_2 laser	Technical specifications – Wavelength 10 600 nm – Power output: 10–20 W Beam delivery – Through an articulated arm with mirrors to a handpiece or colopscope Tissue effect – Strong superficial absorption with carbonization and vaporization of tissue – Cannot be used under water

References

European Project on Monitoring HIV Seroprevalence in a Sentinel Population of STD Patients (1991) Newsletter, no 3, April

Garden JM, O'Banion MK, Shelnitz LS et al (1988) Papillomavirus in the vapor of carbon dioxide laser-treated verrucae. JAMA 259:1199–1202

Hofstetter AG, Frank F (1979) Der Neodym-YAG-Laser in der Urologie. Roche, Basel
Koutsky CA, Galloway DA, Holmes KK (1989) Epidemiology of human papillomavirus
    infection. Epidemiol Rev 10:122–162
Krogh G von (1990) HPV infection of the external genitalia: Clinical aspects and the-
    rapy in dermatovenereology. In: Gross G, Jablonska S, Pfister H, Stegner HE (eds)
    Genital papillomavirus infections. Springer, Berlin Heidelberg New York, pp 156–179
Schneede P (1991) Condylome: Diagnostik und Formen der Therapie. Iatros Urol
    7:30–32
Schneede P, Hofstetter AG (1992) Laserstrahlen zur Behandlung von HPV-Effloreszen-
    zen. Lasermedizin 8:202–205
Schneede P, Kriegmair M, Hofstetter AG (1992) Condylombehandlung mit Neodym-
    YAG-Laser. In: Waidelich W, Waidelich R, Hofstetter AG (eds) Laser in der Medizin.
    Springer, Berlin Heidelberg New York, pp 69–72
Seidl S (1992) Die genitale Papillomvirusinfektion in der gynäkologischen Praxis. In:
    Gross G, Pfister H, Seidl S, Stegner HE (eds) Genitale Infektionen durch Papillom-
    viren. Zuckschwerdt, Munich, pp 59–69
Wickenden C, Steele A, Malcolm AD, Coleman DV (1985) Screening for wart virus
    infection in nommal and abnommal cervical scrapes. Lancet 1:65–67
Zur Hausen H (1987) Papillomaviruses in human cancer. Cancer 59:1692–1696

4.1.2
Penile Carcinoma

K.-H. ROTHENBERGER and A.G. HOFSTETTER

Malignant tumors of the penis are uncommon in Europe and the U.S. compared with India and various African nations. Penile carcinoma is quite rare
in countries where it neonatal circumcision is customary.

Histologically, the majority of penile cancers are squamous cell carcinomas, with scattered reports of metastatic lymphoma and malignant mela-
noma. *Premalignant lesions* consist of balanitis xerotica obliterans, leukoplakia, cutaneous horn, or Buschke-Löwenstein papilloma. *Carcinoma in
situ* may take the form of Queyrat's erythroplasia or Paget's disease of the
penis. The incidence of penile carcinoma in Europe is 0.6–1.3 cases per
100 000 male population.

Conventional treatment options are not only mutilative but are associated with high rates of recurrence (Table 4.2). We have avoided many of

Table 4.2. Recurrence rates of penile carcinoma with conventional treatment methods

Treatment	Recurrence rates (%)	Reference
Local excision	40	Hanash et al. 1970
Partial penectomy (with 2-cm healthy margin)	10	Gursel et al. 1973
Radiotherapy	15	Pointon 1975
Bleomycin	50	Ichikawa 1977
Iridium mold	8	Salaverria et al. 1979

Fig. 4.9. Laser therapy of penile carcinoma (T1, T2, N0, M0; $n=23$). T1, N0, M0, $n=15$: age 59.8 years, average follow-up 7.6 years. T2, N0, M0, $n=8$: age 60.8 years, average follow-up 6.6 years. Five-year disease-free survival rate 92 %, 7-year survival rate more than 83 %

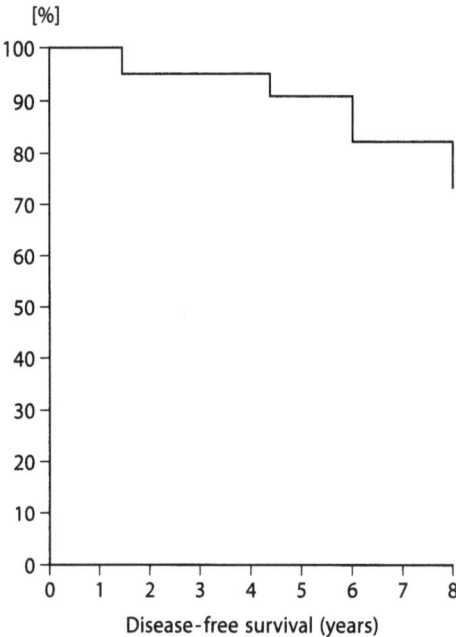

these problems by treating Tis, Ta, T1/(T2), N0, M0 lesions with the Nd:YAG laser, obtaining comparable survival rates with full preservation of penile function and good cosmetic results (Fig. 4.9).

Indications

Laser treatment is appropriate for stage Tis, Ta, T1, T2, N0, M0 carcinomas and various other neoplastic lesions:

- Cavernous hemangioma
- Condylomata acuminata
- Various grades of dysplasia, with or without cornification (grades I–III)
- Bowen's disease
- Queyrat's disease
- Lymphomas, if superficial
- Metastases, if superficial

Preoperative Studies

Inspection and palpation can be supplemented as needed by near-field ultrasound imaging with a high-frequency probe. An intraoperative frozen section can be obtained following circumferential laser denaturation of the tumor margins.

Screening for Metastases

Options include palpation of the inguinal lymph nodes, lymphangiography, CT, fine-needle aspiration biopsy, inguinal lymphadenectomy, and pelvic lymphadenectomy if indicated.

Operative Technique

- A rubber tourniquet is placed around the base of the penis to prevent tumor cell dissemination during the procedure (Fig. 4.10), and a radical circumcision is performed (Fig. 4.11).
- The laser beam is applied circumferentially to about a 0.5- to 1-cm margin surrounding the visible lesion (Fig. 4.12), and a deep biopsy or frozen section specimen is obtained (Fig. 4.13).
- The beam is then swept over the tumor base in linear passes, taking care to avoid skip areas of untreated tissue (Fig. 4.14). The bloodless field produced by the basal tourniquet is very helpful in cases where tumor has been excised from the glans penis or corpora cavernosa. Since the Nd:YAG laser beam is strongly absorbed by blood, it produces carbonization on a bleeding surface, i.e., all the laser energy is absorbed at the surface and cannot penetrate deeply. However, if coagulation is performed in a bloodless field that is also irrigated with sterile saline solution, the beam can penetrate deeply (6–8 mm) and provide effective sealing of the cavernous spaces.

Fig. 4.10. A rubber drain is placed around the base of the penis to function as a tourniquet, and the prepuce is pulled back to expose the carcinoma

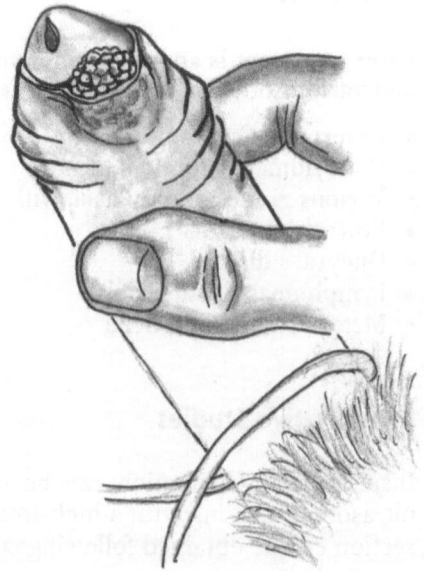

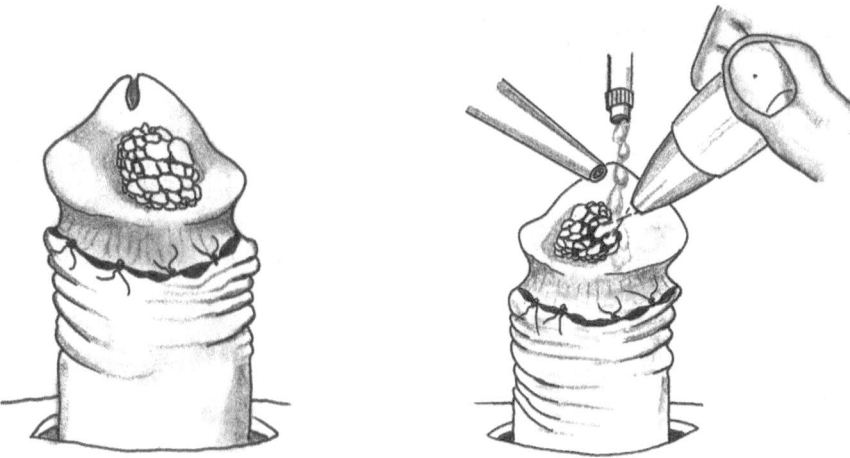

Fig. 4.11 *(left).* Appearance after circumcision and exposure of the penile carcinoma

Fig. 4.12 *(right).* The penile carcinoma is lased with a defocused beam (40 W) from the periphery to the center, including about a 0.5-cm margin. Sterile saline solution is dribbled over the site to promote deep penetration of the laser energy and eliminate the smoke plume

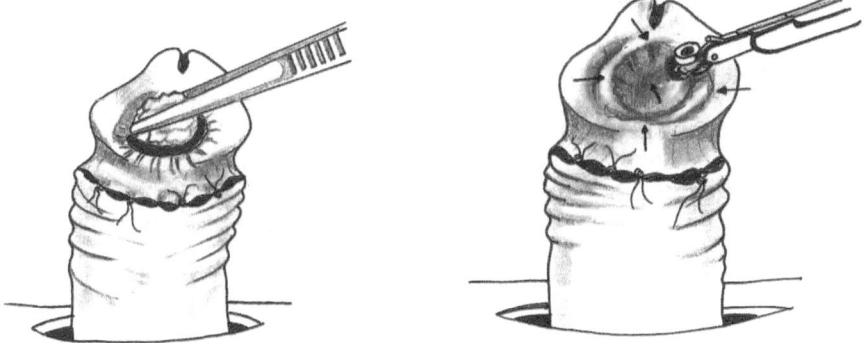

Fig. 4.13 *(left).* Removal of the coagulated tumor

Fig. 4.14 *(right).* Biopsies are taken from the tumor margins at the 3, 6, 9 and 12 o'clock positions and from the center of the tumor crater. The beam is then reapplied to coagulate the entire tumor bed

- A power output of 40–50 W is required.
- After bleeding has been controlled, the tourniquet is released from the base of the penis, and the field is checked for hemostasis.
- The site is covered with sterile gauze and an overlapping Elastoplast bandage.
- Lymphadenectomy is performed if there is *suspicion of metastasis* to the inguinal or pelvic lymph nodes. For this purpose we use a longitudinal incision angled laterally over the center of the inguinal ligament. This incision gives access to the inguinal nodes and can be extended for a pelvic lymphadenectomy.

Advantage of Nd:
YAG Laser Therapy over Conventional Surgical Options

- High efficacy with preservation of penile functions and a good cosmetic result

Follow-up

- Weekly follow-up examinations should be scheduled during the healing period (6–8 weeks). The penis should be bathed daily with a dilute camomile solution or similar cleansing wash.
- The surgical wound should heal leaving a faint scar of variable size, depending on the size of the operative field. If an adequate scar has not formed by 6–8 weeks, the site should be *rebiopsied* and a second laser treatment performed as needed.
- After the tissues have healed, follow-ups should be scheduled at 1-year intervals, and the patient should be seen at 5 years. The patient should be involved in follow-up, as he is likely to notice any ulceration or recurrence of tumor.

Contraindications

- Laser treatment is not suited for advanced tumors that have infiltrated the corpora cavernosa or corpus spongiosum, urethra, prostate, or adjacent organs. The only option in these cases is surgical excision with adequate margins ranging to total penectomy and orchiectomy.
- With metastatic penile carcinoma, the size of the primary tumor determines the suitability of Nd:YAG laser treatment versus penectomy with a trial of systemic chemotherapy (bleomycin, cisplatin, methotrexate, cytokines).

Current radiotherapeutic techniques appear to be unsuitable for the treatment of metastatic penile carcinoma.

Instrumentation

Nd:YAG laser with power output up to 50 W, quartz fiber with focusing handpiece, small surgical tray.

References

Brühl P (1978) Das Peniskarzinom. Dtsch Arztebl 75:1129

Chiari R, Harzmann R (1974) Möglichkeiten der Behandlung von spitzen Kondylomen. Ther Gegenw 113:23

Gursel ED, Gerogountzos C, Uson AC, Melicow MM (1973) Penile cancer: Clinicopathological study of 64 cases. Urology 1:569

Hanash K, Furlow W, Utz D et al (1970) Carcinoma of the penis: a clinical pathological study. J. Urol 104:297

Hofstetter AG, Frank F (1979) Der Neodym-YAG-Laser in der Urologie. Roche, Basel

Hofstetter AG, Staehler G (1977) Das Peniskarzinom. Fortschr Med 95:60

Hofstetter AG, Staehler G, Keiditsch E, Frank F (1978) Lokale Laser-Bestrahlung eines Peniskarzinoms. Fortschr Med 96:369–370

Ichikawa T (1977) Chemotherapy of penile carcinoma. Rec Results Cancer Res 60:140

Pizzocaro G, Pira L (1990) Carcinoma of the penis: diagnosis and treatment. Recent advances in urological cancers. Diagnosis and treatment. Paris, June 27–29, p 251

Pointon RCS (1975) External beam therapy. Proc R Soc Med 68:779

Rothenberger K (1990) Die Behandlung von Peniskarzinomen mit dem Neodym-Yag-Laser in: Zytokine in der urologischen Onkologie. Zuckschwerdt, Munich

Rothenberger K, Hofstetter AG, Geiger M, Bowering R, Frank F (1979) Erfahrungsbericht über die externe Anwendung eines Neodym-Yag-Lasers in der Urologie. Verh Ber Dtsch Ges Urol 31:241

Rothenberger K, Pensel J, Hofstetter AG, Keiditsch E, Stern J (1981) Dosierung der Neodym-Yag-Laserstrahlung zur endovesikalen Anwendung bei Blasentumoren – tierexperimentelle Untersuchungen. Urologie A 20:310

Salaverria JC, Hope-Stone HF, Paris AMJ, Molland EA, Blandy JP (1979) Conservative treatment of carcinoma of the penis. Br J Urol 51:32

Seer Program (1974–1986) Cancer statistics reviews 1973–87. National Cancer Institute, Bethesda, NIH publication no 90–2789

Skinner DG, Leadbetter WF, Kelley SB (1972) The surgical management of squamous cell carcinoma of the penis. J Urol 107:272

Staehler G (1981) Die externe Anwendung von Neodym-Yag-Laserstrahlung in der Urologie. Urologe A 20:323

4.2
Urethra

4.2.1
Laser Treatment of Urethral Strictures

P. Schneede, R. Klammert, and A.G. Hofstetter

The standard primary treatment for urethral strictures, internal urethrotomy, fails in approximately 20 % of cases, even when repeated, due to recurrent stricture formation (Smith et al. 1983). The postoperative strictures in these cases may be more severe than the original lesions (Merkle 1991). To obviate the need for an open urethroplasty in patients with recurrent strictures, attempts have been made since the mid-1970 s to treat these lesions with laser irradiation (Bülow et al. 1979; Hofstetter and Frank 1979). Today, given the great variety of laser systems and delivery methods that are available, a distinction must be drawn between coagulating lasers with high thermal activity (Smith 1991; Smith and Dixon 1984) and cutting lasers with low thermal activity (Malloy et al. 1990; Merkle 1991; Wagner et al. 1992).

Etiology

Studies on the etiology of urethral strictures (Nöske et al. 1992) have shown that the majority of benign strictures are secondary to iatrogenic manipulations of the urethra.

- Iatrogenic (65 %)
  - Urethrotomy
  - Other surgical procedures (e.g., transurethral resection, TUR)
  - Catheterization or dilatation
  - Urethrocystoscopy
- Infections (14 %)
- Trauma (8 %)
- Anomalies (1 %)
- Unknown (12 %)

Any incision of the urethra can create a stimulus for the formation of intraluminal granulations leading to excessive scarring and recurrent stricturing (Merkle 1991). Treatment and outcome are critically influenced by the degree of circumferential luminal narrowing of the urethra and by the length of the strictured area. Long segmental strictures have a significantly poorer prognosis. This is also true if urethral ultrasound demonstrates peristrictural scarring in addition to the lumen-reducing scar tissue (Merkle 1991).

Indications

The curative use of laser urethrotomy is appropriate for:

- Primary and recurrent penile urethral strictures
- Bladder neck contracture
- Anastomotic stricture following radical prostatectomy
- Urethral valves

Preoperative Studies

Uroflowmetry, urethrocystography, voiding cystourethrography, urethrocystoscopy, urethral ultrasound.

Operative Technique

Two types of laser system are used, each with different actions and modes of operation.

- Lasers with high thermal activity (e.g., argon laser, Rothauge et al. 1981).
  - Used in noncontact mode
  - Thermal lasers are unsuited for the penile urethra but can be used on the bradytrophic tissue of the membranous urethra (Gilbert and Beckert 1993) and on urethral valves (Ehrlich et al. 1987).
  - Deep tissue penetration (e.g., 4–8 mm for the Nd:YAG laser) with thermal necrosis and coagulation (Keiditsch 1981).
- Lasers for contact cutting.
  - Laser fiber cuts on contact with tissue.
  - Well suited for the penile urethra.
  - Shallow penetration (e.g., 0.03 mm for the excimer laser), no deep coagulative necrosis.

Methods of Application

- Lasers with high thermal activity are reserved for highly selected indications.
  - The beam is moved over the bradytrophic tissue in a linear pattern, without contact, until the tissue whitens.
  - The lased necrotic tissue is sloughed.
  - Precise laser application is important. Overirradition of neighboring tissue can incite heavy peristrictural fibrosis and recurrent stricturing.
- Lasers for contact cutting (Fig. 4.15).
  - The incision basically follows the urethrotomy technique of Sachse (1974), using a cutting speed of 0.2–0.3 mm/s (Wagner et al. 1992).
  - Instead of a cold knife incision at 12 o'clock, a notch is made at that position with the contact tip of the laser fiber.

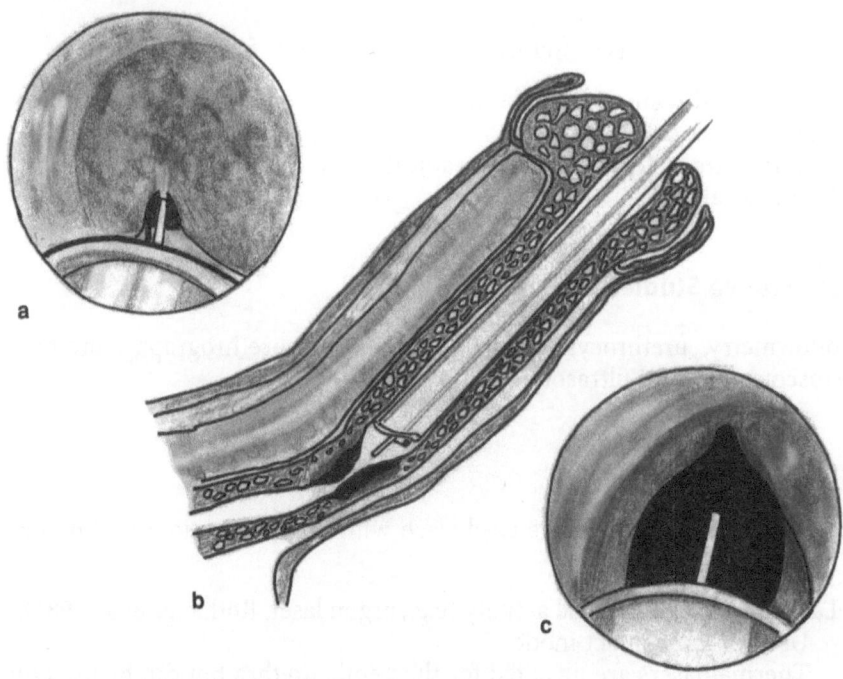

Fig. 4.15. a Dorsal incision with the Nd:YAG laser (20 W) for treatment of a penile urethral stricture. **b** Penile urethral stricture (schematic view). **c** Condition following laser incision of the urethral stricture at 12 o'clock

- There is little tissue penetration of the beam, which produces a narrow zone of coagulation but effectively prevents bleeding from opened vessels at the margin of the incision.
- As notching of the stricture proceeds, the laser fiber is visually guided through the cystoscope using an Albarran deflector.
- Notching of the stricture at multiple sites (4, 8, and 12 o'clock) has proved particularly effective for the treatment of bladder neck contractures and anastomotic strictures after radical prostatectomy (Gilbert and Beckert 1993) in the proximal portion of the urethra.
- With high-grade strictures, a guidewire should be used in conjunction with the laser urethrotomy.

Advantages of the Laser over Conventional Treatments: Minimal Invasiveness

- Alternative treatments for urethral strictures:
  - Internal urethrotomy (after Sachse or Otis)
  - Dilatation

- Wall stent implantation
- Open urethroplastic procedures
- The advantages mainly apply to lasers used for contact cutting:
  - Superficial coagulation prevents bleeding from opened vessels, thereby reducing the tendency for postoperative adhesion of the cut edges.
  - Since the incisions are bloodless, there is no need for routine bladder catheterization. This can shorten the hospital stay and may permit the surgery to be carried out as an outpatient procedure.

Follow-up

- Most recurrent strictures form during the first 6 months after surgery. Follow-up examinations during this period should include uroflowmetry, urethrocystography, and repeated urethral ultrasound examinations as required.
- Larger studies are needed to determine whether dilatations can be dispensed with after laser urethrotomy.

Contraindications

Lasers with high thermal activity should be used only in highly selected cases. These lasers should not be used in the penile urethra due to the potential for postoperative peristrictural fibrosis and the high incidence of recurrent strictures.

Instrumentation

Below, laser systems that produce noncontact coagulation of strictured tissue are contrasted with laser systems that are suitable for contact cutting without producing a deep thermal effect.

Laser Systems for Urethrotomy

- Laser systems with high thermal activity:
  - Nd:YAG laser, CO_2 laser
  - Argon laser
- Lasers for contact cutting:
  - Excimer laser
  - Erbium laser
  - Nd:YAG Fibertome
  - KTP laser
  - Holmium:YAG laser

Fig. 4.16 Distal laser urethrotomy is performed by withdrawing the laser fiber along the scalpel guide of the open urethrotome. Coexisting HPV lesions in the path of the beam are also destroyed

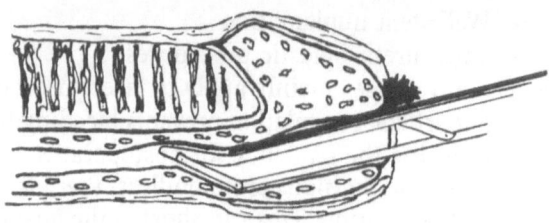

A common feature of all these systems is that the laser energy can be delivered through quartz fibers, and the lasers can be used inside the urethra while water irrigation is applied. The laser fiber is introduced through an endoscope, and an Albarran deflector may be used for greater accuracy of beam projection.

If meatal stenosis coexists with HPV lesions (see also Sect. 4.1), we use a pediatric Otis urethrotome to guide the laser fiber, which is drawn along the scalpel groove in the urethrotome at the 12 o'clock position (Fig. 4.16). This provides a straight cut of uniform depth that incises the stricture and also destroys the HPV lesions in the area of the cut (Schneede et al.).

References

Bülow H, Bülow U, Frohmüller HGW (1979) Transurethral laser urethrotomy in man: preliminary report. J Urol 121:286–287

Ehrlich RM, Shanberg A, Fine RV (1987) Neodymium:YAG laser ablation of posterior urethral valves. J Urol 138:959–962

Gilbert P, Beckert R (1993) Post-prostatectomy stricture of the membranous urethra and its removal by Nd:YAG laser coagulation. Lasermedizin 9:90–93

Hofstetter AG, Frank F (1979) Der Neodym-YAG-Laser in der Urologie. Roche, Basel

Keiditsch E (1981) Histologische Grundlagen der endovesikalen Neodym:YAG-Laser-Bestrahlung. Urologe A 20:300–304

Malloy TR, Turek PJ, Cendrone M, Carpienello VC, Wein AJ (1990) KTP/532 laser ablation of urethral strictures. J Urol 143:403A

Merkle W (1991) Laserinzisionen zur Behandlung rezidivierender Harnröhrenstenosen des Mannes. Lasermedizin 7:91–95

Noske HD, Mikhael-Beaupain A, Rothauge CF (1992) Der Argonlaser und die Harnröhrenstriktur. In: Merkle W, Haupt (eds) Moderne Methoden der Sonographie und Lasertherapie in der Urologie. Biermann, Zülpich

Rothauge CF, Noske HD, Kraushaar J (1981) Erfahrungen mit der Argon-Laserapplikation bei urologischen Erkrankungen. Urologe A 20:333–339

Rothenberger KG, Hofstetter AG (1994) Lasertherapie des Peniskarzinoms. Urologe A 33:231–234

Sachse H (1974) Zur Behandlung der Harnröhrenstriktur: Die transurethrale Schlitzung unter Sicht mit scharfem Schnitt. Fortschr Med 92:12–15

Schneede P, Fink H-U, Muschter R, Hofstetter AG (1996) Laser-Urethrotomie zur Behandlung von Strikturen und koinzidenten HPV-Infektionen der distalen Harnröhre. Lasermedizin (in press)

Smith JA Jr (1991) Urological laser surgery. Hospimedica 9:50–55

Smith JA Jr, Dixon JA (1984) Neodymium:YAG laser treatment of benign urethral strictures. J Urol 131:1080–1081
Smith PJB, Roberts JBM, Ball AJ, Kaisary AV (1983) Long-term results of optical urethrotomy. Br J Urol 55:689–700
Wagner W, Bauer H, Altwein JE, Schneider W (1992) Die Behandlung rezidivierender Harnröhrenstrikturen mittels Photoablation durch Excimer-Laser. In: Merkle W, Haupt (eds) Moderne Methoden der Sonographie und Lasertherapie in der Urologie. Bierrnann, Zülpich

4.3
Bladder

A.G. HOFSTETTER

The neodymium:YAG laser produces a deep, homogeneous coagulating effect that can selectively destroy benign and malignant lesions of the bladder wall (polyps, hemangiomas, endometriotic deposits, carcinomas, metastases, schistosomal lesions, interstitial and radiation cystitis, arteritis nodosa, etc.)

This surgery requires a power output of 20–40 W, so special care must be taken during laser use on the posterior bladder wall due to the risk of bowel perforation. With larger lesions, pelviscopic monitoring should be performed during the laser surgery (Fig. 4.17).

4.3.1
Bladder Cancer

The Nd:YAG laser can destroy bladder tumors by both interstitial and non-contact application with concomitant sealing of blood vessels and lymphatics (Halldørsson and Langerhole 1978; Hofstetter 1986, 1988, 1992; Hofstetter and Frank 1979). When the proper application technique is used (perpendicular beam angle, fluid distention), Nd:YAG photoirradiation produces a deep, well-defined, homogeneous zone of tissue necrosis that encompasses the full thickness of the bladder wall (Fig. 4.18).

Indications (Fig. 4.19)

- Curative: Ta–T2 (3), N0, M0 lesions
- Palliative: T3–T4, N1–4, Mx/M1 lesions
- Carcinoma in situ, severe dysplasia (Photodynamic diagnosis and therapy are indicated for multiple confluent lesions; photodynamic diagnosis and Nd:YAG or diode laser treatment are indicated for isolated lesions.)

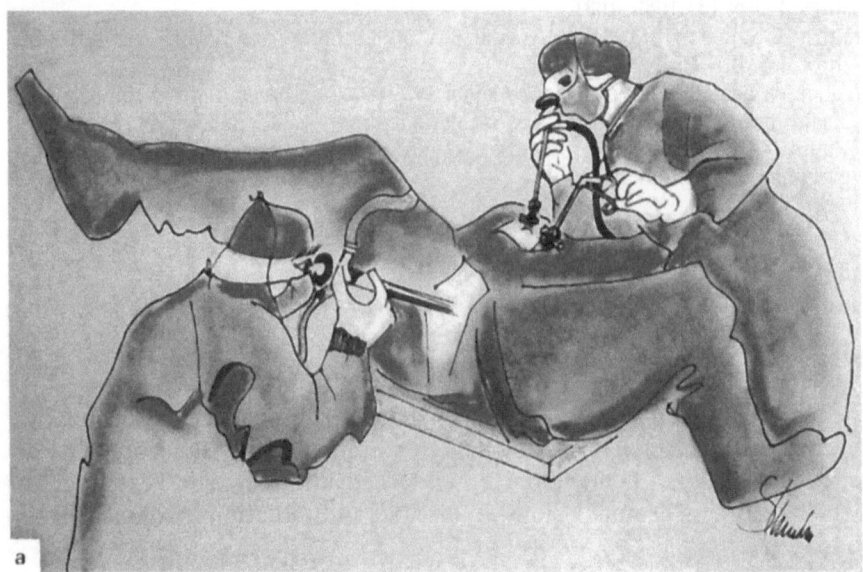

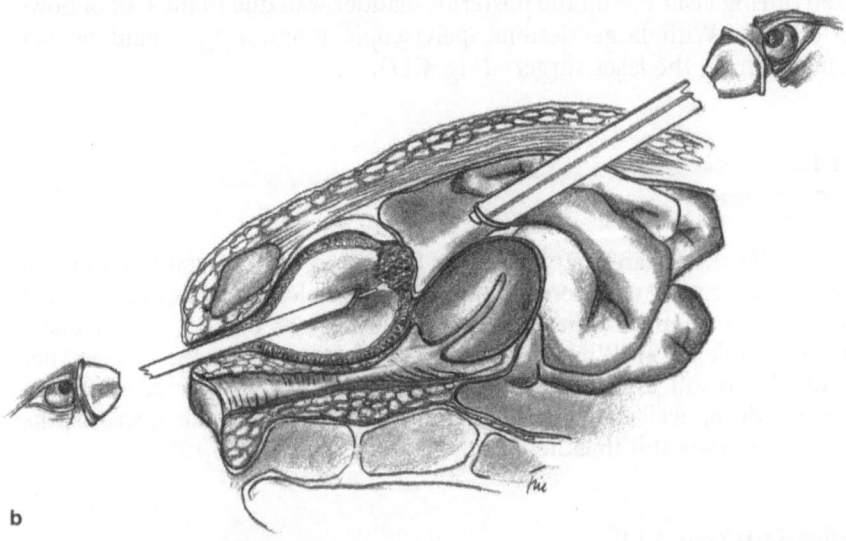

Fig. 4.17 a, b. Endoscopic laser treatment of a carcinoma of the posterior bladder wall (40 W), with laparoscopic monitoring

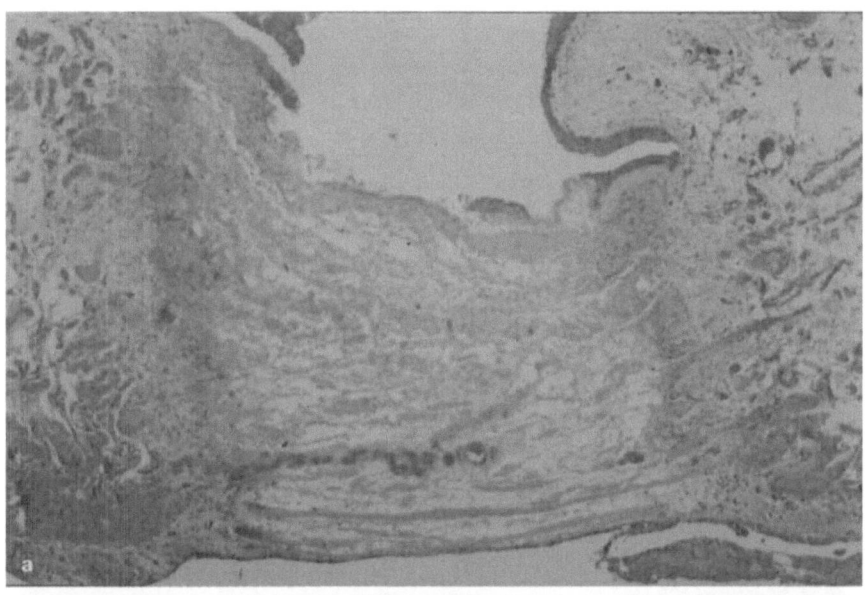

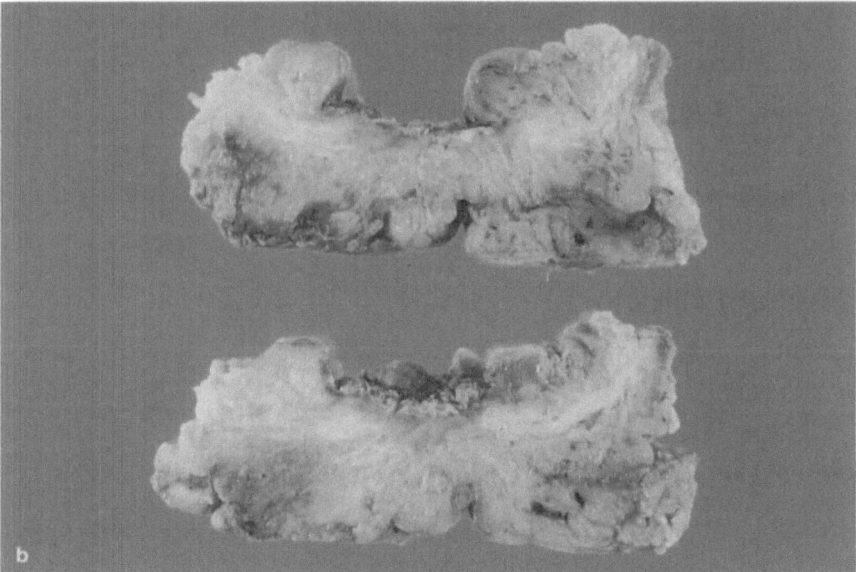

Fig. 4.18. a Homogeneous, full-thickness necrosis of the bladder wall produced by Nd:YAG laser irradiation in the rabbit. **b** Full-thickness bladder wall necrosis after the Nd:YAG laser irradiation of a human bladder cancer (sagittal sections). (From Keiditsch et al. 1977, 1986)

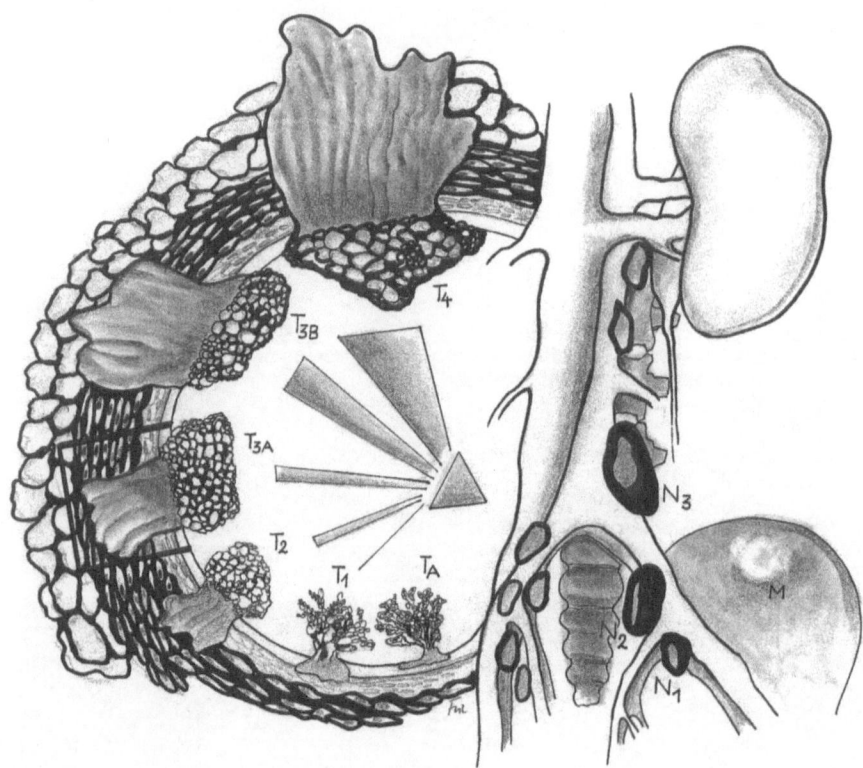

Fig. 4.19. TNM stages of bladder carcinoma

Preoperative Studies

Intravenous urography, lavage cytology, cystoscopy, and selective biopsy aided by photodynamic diagnosis.

Screening for Metastases

Pelvic and abdominal CT, chest radiograph, open or laparoscopic lymphadenectomy, bone scan, bone marrow biopsy, CT-guided lymph node biopsy.

Operative Technique

- Laser power output: 20–40 W, depending on bladder distention, bladder wall thickness, and exposure time (Fig. 4.20).
- Depth of penetration: 0.4–0.8 cm, although electron microscopic studies have demonstrated thermal effects as deep as 1.2–1.6 cm (Lehmann et al. 1988).

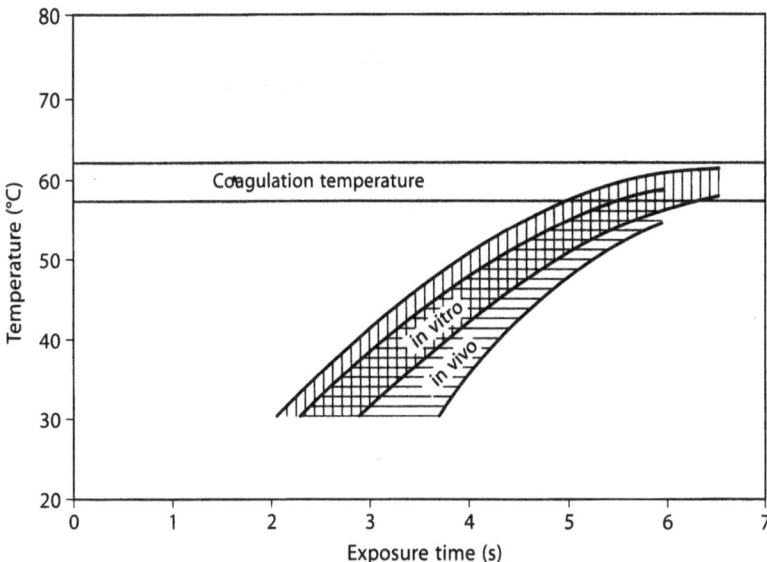

Fig. 4.20. Temperature distribution in the human posterior bladder wall (bladder wall thickness 7–10 mm) in vivo and in vitro during Nd:YAG laser irradiation (45 W, 2–6 s, irradiated area approximately 3 mm in diameter). (From Pensel et al. 1981)

- Penetration of the laser energy is *decreased* by a severely inflamed or richly vascularized bladder mucosa, by gas distention of the bladder, and by bleeding or blood-tinged irrigation fluid.
- Penetration of the laser energy is *increased* by fluid distention of the bladder.
- Bladder wall thickness: 0.4–0.7 cm in adults with 200 ml fluid distention.
- Bladder wall thickness may be decreased in patients who have had previous bladder surgery.
- Caution should be exercised during laser treatment of the posterior bladder wall.
  The laser treatment of large areas of the posterior bladder wall should be monitored laparoscopically, especially in previously operated patients, as there is a risk of perforating bowel that is adherent to the bladder wall (Fig. 4.17).

Application Technique (Fig. 4.22a–d)

- The bladder is distended with 0.9 % NaCl solution (200 ml in adults).
- The focused laser beam is applied to the tumor base in linear passes, then if possible the beam is swept around the circumference of the tumor to create a 0.5–1 cm whitened margin ("Spanish collar") completely surrounding the lesion (Hofstetter and Frank 1979, 1981, 1985; Meier et al.

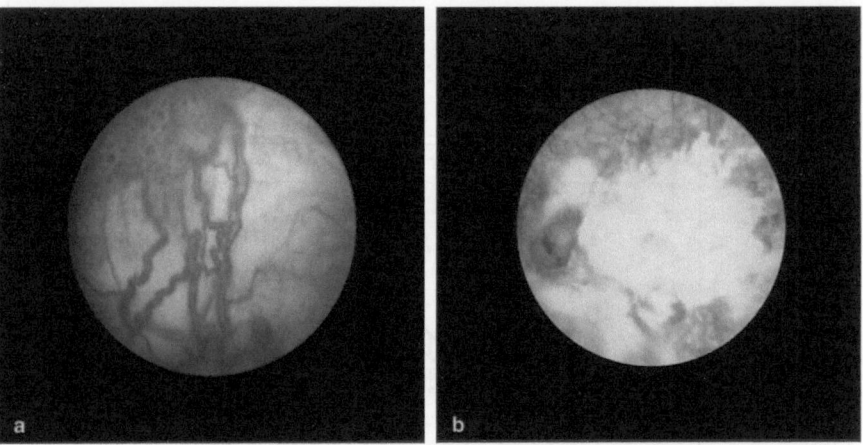

Fig. 4.21. a Typical appearance of bladder tumor vessels prior to laser treatment.
b Appearance of the vessels after Nd:YAG laser treatment. These feeding vessels are
important as they mark the location of satellite lesions that are often overlooked

1985; Spitzenpfeil et al. 1989; Staehler and Hofstetter 1979). If the tumor
cannot be completely encircled, it is sufficient to treat one-half to three-
quarters of the circumference of the tumor base. Then the laser fiber is
applied interstitially (Fig. 4.23c); this may be performed as an alternative
to, or in conjunction with, line-by-line irradiation of the exophytic portion. This process destroys the central vascular supply of the tumor and
prevents the heavy, troublesome bleeding that often occurs during the
resection of large exophytic tumors (Fig. 4.23a–c).
- Special attention is given to the tumor vessels (Fig. 4.21). They should be
  selectively destroyed by moving the laser beam along each vessel. These
  vessels are also useful for defining the extent of the main tumor and
  locating satellite lesions.
- For tumors with an exophytic portion that is cherry-size or smaller
  (Fig. 4.22a–d):
  - The Nd:YAG laser beam is applied to the tumor base and surrounding
    tissues (Fig. 4.22b) and to the main tumor mass (Fig. 4.22c).
  - The lased tumor is removed with a biopsy forceps (Fig. 4.22d).
  - The laser is reapplied to the tumor *margins*, creating a 0.5- to 1.0-cm
    zone of coagulation.
- For tumors with a larger than cherry-size exophytic portion (Fig. 4.23a–f):
  - The tumor base and surrounding tissues are lased, and the tumor
    mass is treated interstitially and/or with noncontact linear passes of
    the beam.
  - The lased tumor area is resected (Fig. 4.23d).
  - The Nd:YAG laser is reapplied to the tumor margins and base
    (Fig. 4.23 f), sealing any blood vessels and lymphatics that have been
    opened by the TUR.

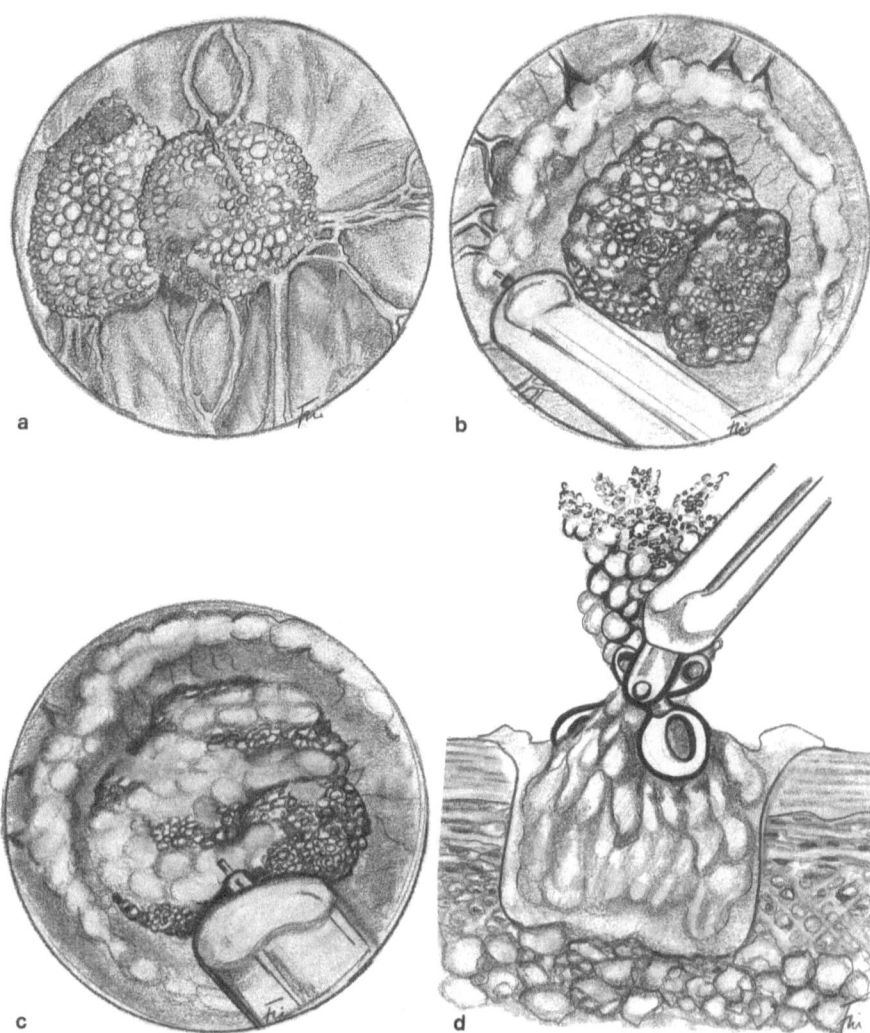

Fig. 4.22. a Typical bladder tumor with feeding vessels (schematic drawing). **b** The feeding vessels are sealed, and the tumor margin is coagulated to form a whitened "Spanish collar" 0.5–1 cm wide. **c** The exophytic portion of the mass is destroyed with linear passes of the Nd:YAG laser. **d** The laser-coagulated tumor is removed (lateral view)

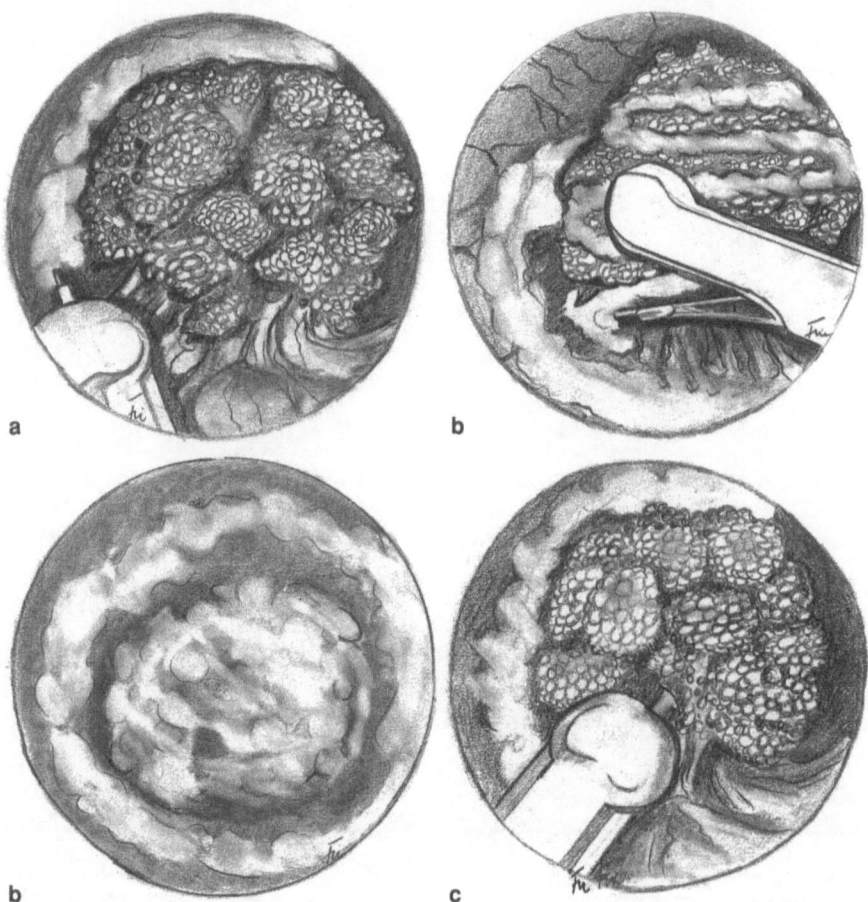

Fig. 4.23. a The Nd:YAG laser fiber is moved in a semicircular pattern around the base of a large bladder tumor. **b** The exophytic portion of the tumor is coagulated with linear passes using noncontact technique. **b'** Care is taken to avoid skip areas of untreated tumor. **c** Fiber placement for interstitial laser treatment. **d-f** see p. 75

Advantages of Nd:YAG Laser Treatment over TUR

- The Nd:YAG laser produces primary, noncontact sealing of blood vessels and lymphatics. This avoids mechanical destruction of the lamina propria and vascular disruption caused by TUR and the associated risks of tumor cell dissemination (Page et al. 1978; Soloway and Martens 1980; Weldon and Soloway 1975).
- Since the Nd:YAG laser seals off the central blood supply of the tumor, there is little if any bleeding during resection of the exophytic mass.
- An added benefit is that the Nd:YAG laser sterilizes all residual cancer cells in the irradiated area.

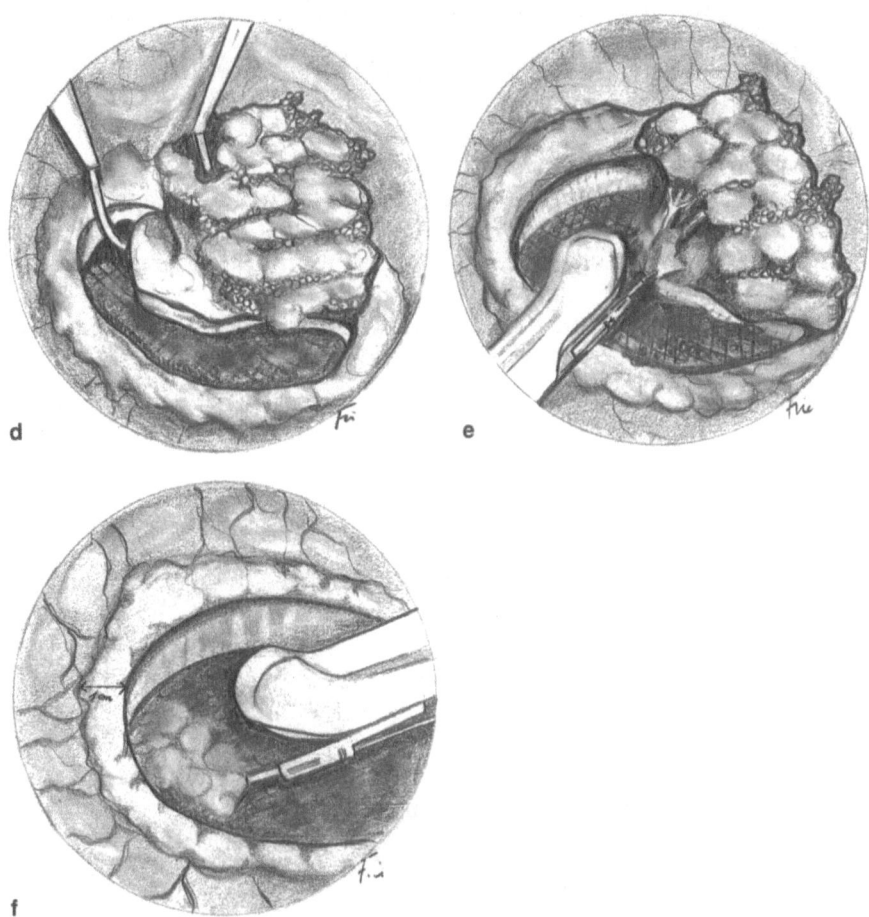

Fig. 4.23 *(continued).* **d** The treated tumor masses are removed with a TUR cutting loop or biopsy forceps. *Special case:* Very large exophytic masses can be lased and removed piecemeal (**e, f**). After the lased portions have been removed with the cutting loop or forceps, the beam is reapplied to the residual tumor (**e**). **f** After all lased tumor has been removed, the tumor base and margins are irradiated

Follow-up

- A cystoscopic follow-up examination is scheduled 4 weeks postoperatively. Photodynamic diagnosis also may be performed if desired (see Chap. 5).
- Cystoscopic follow-ups are scheduled every 3 months during the first year, and photodynamic diagnosis is performed every 6 months.
- Six-month visits are scheduled after the first year.
- After 4 years, cystoscopic examinations are performed annually and may be supplemented by photodynamic diagnosis.

- Recurrent tumor is managed and followed in the same way as the primary tumor.
- For well-differentiated carcinomas, staging is performed every 6 months for 1 year, then annual follow-ups are scheduled (CT, bone scans, bone marrow biopsies as required). Cystoscopic follow-ups are performed every 6 months for 3 years and once a year thereafter.
- For moderately and poorly differentiated carcinomas, staging is performed every 6 months for 2 years, with annual follow-ups thereafter. Cystoscopic follow-ups with cytological examination are performed every 6 months for 5 years.
- For T1b to T4 infiltrating tumors with no CT evidence of lymph node involvement, laparoscopic pelvic lymphadenectomy should be performed.

Contraindications

- Contracted bladder
- Multiple carcinomas in situ (poorly differentiated), D_2 or D_3 dysplasia
- "Bulky disease"

Instrumentation

The Multiscope (a laser endoscope designed by Hofstetter, Baumgartner, and Kriegmair and manufactured by Storz):

- For the photodynamic detection and Nd:YAG laser treatment of tumor sites
- For photodynamic diagnosis and TUR

References

Benson RC (1986) Integral photoradiation therapy of multifocal bladder tumors. Eur Urol 12 [Suppl 1]:47–53

Frank F (1979) Der Nd-YAG-Laser. Thesis, Universitat

Halldørsson T, Langerholc J (1978) Thermodynamic analysis of laser irradiation of biological tissue. Appl Optics 17:3948–3950

Hofstetter AG (1986) Treatment of urological tumors by Nd-YAG laser. Eur Urol 12 [Suppl 1]:21–24

Hofstetter AG (1988) Laserkoagulationstherapie des Harnblasenkarzinoms. In: Schuler J, Hofstetter AG (eds) Endourologie. Thieme, Stuttgart, p 261

Hofstetter AG (1992) Application of lasers in bladder cancer. Semin Surg Oncol 8:214–216

Hofstetter AG, Böwering R, Frank F, Keidtisch E, Pensel J, Rothenberger KH, Staehler G (1980) DHW 105:1492–1494

Hofstetter AG, Frank F (1979) Ein neues Laser-Endoskop zur Bestrahlung von Blasentumoren. Fortschr Med 97:232–234

Hofstetter AG, Frank F (1979) Der Neodym-YAG-Laser in der Urologie. Roche, Basel
Hofstetter AG, Frank F (1981) Endoscopic Nd:YAG laser application for destroying bladder tumors. Eur Urol 7:278–279
Hofstetter AG, Frank F (1985) Laser treatment of bladder tumors: experimental and clinical resuluts. In: Smith JA Jr (ed) Lasers in urology surgery. Year Book, Chicago
Jocham D, Schmiedt E, Staehler G (1985) Photodynamic laser therapy of multifocal bladder carcinoma using hematoporphyrin derivative (HPD) as a tumor photosensitizer. XXth Congr Int Soc Urol, Vienna
Keiditsch E (1986) Morphological fundamentals in the treatment of tumors with the Nd:YAG laser. Eur Urol 12 [Suppl 1]:12–16
Keiditsch E, Langer R, Staehler G, Hofstetter AG (1977) Morphologische Veränderungen an der Kaninchenharnblase nach Laserbestrahlung. Verh Dtsch Ges Pathol 61:367–369
Lehmann R, Meier H, Willital GH (1988) Veränderungen intra- und extrazellulärer Strukturen nach Nd:YAG Laser-Resektion. Laser Med Surg 4:116–119
Meier U, Hofstetter AG, Pflüger H (1985) Effects of intravesical instillation of mitomycin after endoscopic treatment with TUR or laser and recurrence rate of bladder tumors. XXth Congr Int Soc Urol, Vienna
Page BH, Levison UB, Corwen MP (1978) The site of recurrence of noninfiltrating bladder tumors. Br J Urol 50:237–238
Pensel J, Hofstetter AG, Frank F et al (1981) Temporal and spatial temperature profile of the bladder serosa in intravesical Nd:YAG laser irradiation. Eur Urol 7:298–300
Pensel J, Hofstetter AG, Keiditsch E, Staehler G (1979) Wärmeleitung auf der Blasenrückwand während der endoskopischen Laserbestrahlung. 3rd International Congress on Laser Surgery, Graz
Soloway MS, Martens S (1980) Urothelial receptibility to tumor cell implantation: influence of catheterization. Cancer 46:1158–1163
Spitzenpfeil E, Hofstetter AG, Reis M, Muschter R (1989) Nd:YAG-Laser bei infiltrierenden Blasentumoren. Fortschr Med 107:548–550
Staehler G, Hofstetter AG (1979) Transurethral laser irradiation of urinary bladder tumors. Eur Urol 5:64–69
Weldon TE, Soloway MS (1975) Susceptibility of urothelium to neoplastic cellular implantation. Urology 5:824–827
Zimmermann J, Stern J, Frank F, Kreiditsch E, Hofstetter AG (1984) Interception of lymphatic drainage by Nd:YAG laser irradiation in the rat urinary bladder. Laser Surg Mediastinosc 4:167–172

4.3.2
Urinary Schistosomiasis (Fig. 4.24)

The worm *Schistosoma haematobium*, a digenetic trematode, lives in the prostatovesical venous plexus. The females lay their eggs mainly in the subepithelial and interstitial layers of the bladder. The egg deposits incite a local inflammatory reaction with infiltration of round cells, monocytes, eosinophils, and giant cells that form tubercles and nodules. Later there is scar formation, ulceration, and epithelial metaplasia that may progress to squamous cell carcinoma. Secondary infection of the urinary tract is a frequent complication. The trapped dead eggs are not extruded into the bladder lumen; they calcify and form sheets of subepithelial calcified layers in the area of the ureter, bladder, and seminal vesicles.

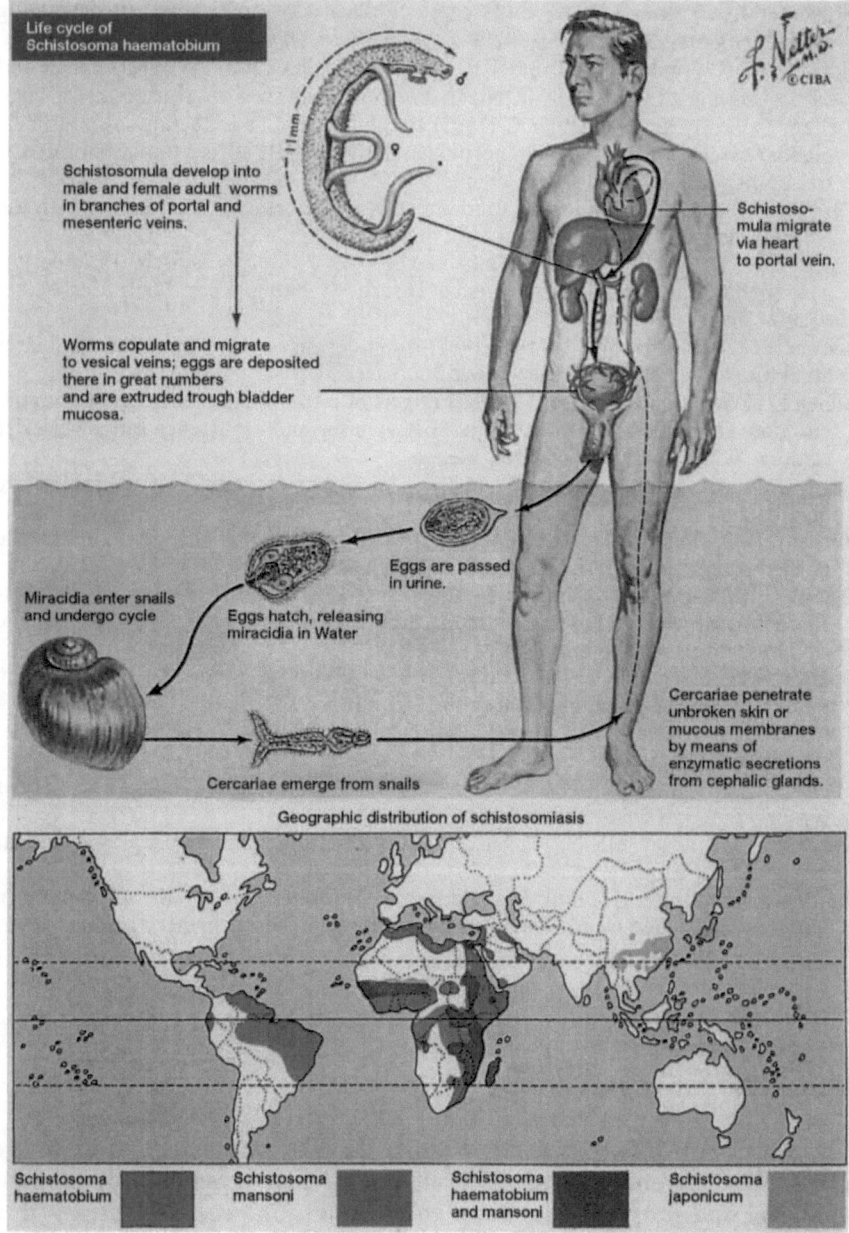

Fig. 4.24. The life cycle of *Schistosoma haematobium* (from the Ciba Collection)

Fig. 4.25. Schistosomal tubercles in the bladder mucosa

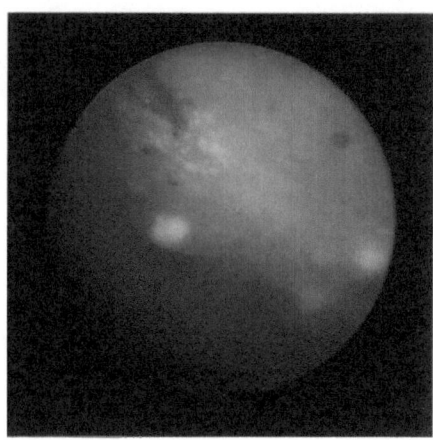

These pathophysiological changes are marked by typical cystoscopic findings:

- Initial stage:
  - Tubercles (Fig. 4.25)
  - Nodules
  - Polyps
- Early changes:
  - "Sandy patches" and ground-glass areas of mucosa that lack a normal vascular pattern
  - Acute and chronic ulcers
  - Glandular and cystic cystitis
- Late complications:
  - Contracted bladder
  - Bladder outlet obstruction
  - Leukoplakia
  - Carcinoma in situ
  - Invasive carcinoma

Indications

All acute and chronic schistosomal bladder lesions are treatable with the Nd:YAG laser, except in a severely contracted bladder. With a bladder neck contracture, Nd:YAG laser incisions should be made at the 5, 7, and 12 o'clock positions. Localized calcifications and calcified schistosomal ova can be fragmented with a laser lithotriptor.

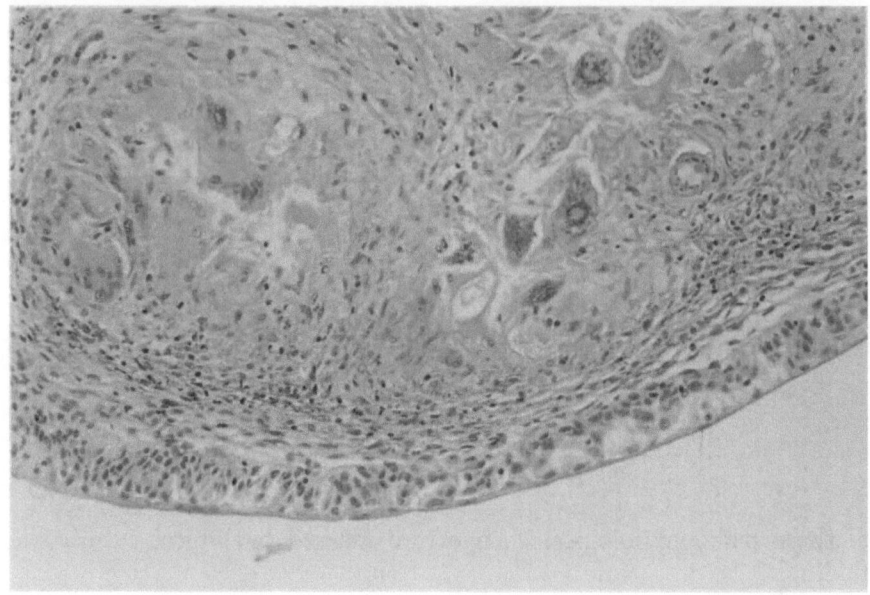

Fig. 4.26. Typical histological appearance of schistosomal eggs in the bladder mucosa. H&E stain

Preoperative Studies

Intravenous urography, detection of eggs in the urine, urethrocystoscopy, and bladder wall biopsy (Fig. 4.26).

Screening for Metastases

Same as for bladder cancer (see Sect. 4.3.1).

Operative Technique (Fig. 4.27)

- Grossly visible lesions are destroyed with linear passes of the Nd:YAG laser. (Photodynamic diagnosis and therapy should be performed if they prove to be as useful for schistosomal lesions as for bladder cancer.)
- Power output: 20–40 W.
- Noncontact destruction of the schistosomal lesions (including eggs).

Cystoscopic Follow-up

- Four weeks after laser surgery
- Then every 6 months for 2 years

Fig. 4.27. Nd:YAG laser treatment (20 W) of inflammatory and ulcerative schistosomal lesions of the bladder mucosa

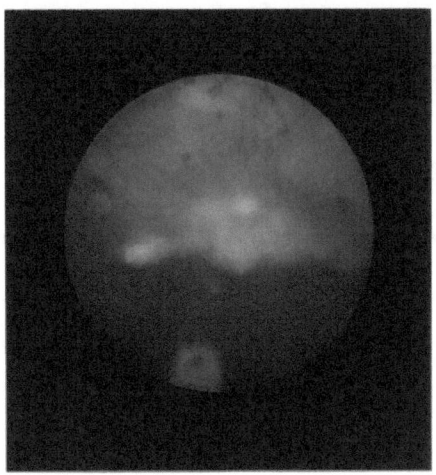

Contraindications

- Severely contracted bladder
- Multiple foci of carcinoma or carcinoma in situ
- Multiple foci of dysplasia (D_2, D_3)

4.3.3
Interstitial Cystitis (Hunner's Ulcer, Submucous Fibrosis)

Mainly a disease of middle-aged women, interstitial cystitis is characterized by fibrosis of the bladder wall with a progressive loss of bladder capacity leading to pollakisuria, urinary urgency, and pelvic pain.

The cause of interstitial cystitis is unknown but may relate to an autoimmune collagen disorder. The primary change is fibrosis in the deeper layers of the bladder. The bladder endothelium is thinned, especially at the dome, and small ulcerations or tears of the mucosa may be found in this area. In severe cases there may be involvement of the bladder outlet or ureterovesical junction, leading to vesicoureteral reflux and possibly hydronephrosis.

During *endoscopic examination*, the patient experiences typical suprapubic pain as the bladder is slowly filled. The bladder mucosa may look fairly normal, but punctate hemorrhages or larger petechial areas often appear as bladder distention is increased. Ulcers are rarely seen.

Indications

Nd:YAG laser treatment of mucosal lesions is appropriate for patients with pain, urgency, and ulceration.

Preoperative Studies

Intravenous urography, cystoscopy, and bladder biopsies.

Operative Technique

- Suspicious areas and ulcers are treated with linear passes of the laser fiber.
- After the procedure patients experience an immediate, dramatic relief of symptoms.
- The power output is 20–25 W, and a total dose of up to 30 000 J may be delivered in one session.
  (Research is currently being carried out to assess the potential efficacy of photodynamic diagnosis and treatment for this disease.)

Follow-up

If pain recurs, the patient should undergo repeat cystoscopy, and additional laser treatment is performed as needed.

Contraindications

- A severely contracted bladder contraindicates laser therapy. In these extreme cases a bladder expansion procedure or bladder reconstruction should be performed.

References

Dann T, Pensel J, Hofstetter AG (1988) Bilharziose – Ursache einer therapierefraktaren Zystitis? Einsatz des Nd:YAG-Lasers. 30. Tag. Verein Norddeutsche Urologen, Hamburg

Dunshee C, Shanberg AM (1993) Benign diseases of the bladder. In: Smith JA, Stein BS, Benson RC (eds) Lasers in urological surgery. Mosby, St. Louis, pp 107–112

Hammouda HMM (1993) Use of Nd:YAG laser in treatment of benign bilharzial lesions of urinary bladder. Thesis, Assiut University, Egypt

Hofstetter AG, Frank F (1984) Nd:YAG-Laser in der Urologie. Med Foc 3:2

Hofstetter AG (1986) Unspezifische und spezifische Entzündungen des Urogenitaltraktes. In: Hofstetter AG, Eisenberger F (eds) Urologie für die Praxis. Bergmann, Munich, p 108

Hofstetter AG (1989) Laseranwendung schafft neue Perspektiven. Fortschr Med 107/26:545–546

Pensel J, Dann T, Hofstetter AG (1986) Schistosmiasis as a cause of painful urogenital syndrome. IX International Congress of Infections and Parasitic Disease, Munich

4.4
Ureter

A.G. HOFSTETTER

4.4.1
Ureteral Tumors

Indications

- Solitary kidney (functional or anatomic)
- Renal failure
- Increased risk of recurrent cancer, as in renal transplant recipients (immunosuppression!)
- Bilateral tumor involvement
- Endemic nephropathy
- Increased cancer risk due to phenacetin abuse, heavy exposure to aromatic hydrocarbons, etc
- Curative treatment of Ta–T2, N0, M0 tumors (Fig. 4.28). In advanced cases, laser treatment can be used palliatively in conjunction with chemotherapy (e.g., MVEC)

Preoperative Studies

Intravenous urography, lavage cytology prior to retrograde ureteropyelography or ureteroscopy and biopsy; if positive: screen for metastases.

Screening for Metastases

- CT (pelvic, abdominal), bone scan, bone marrow biopsy, biplane chest radiographs.

Operative Technique

- Ureteroscopy:
  - The ureteroscope is inserted to the tumor site, with or without a guidewire, and the site is inspected using 0° and 30° telescopes. All of the tumor must be visualized (Fig. 4.29).
  - The tumor base is selectively coagulated with individual Nd:YAG laser pulses (20–30 W) of 1–2 s duration (Fig. 4.30).
  - The lased tumor is removed with a rigid or flexible biopsy forceps (Fig. 4.31).
  - The beam is reapplied to the tumor area (Fig. 4.32).

Caution: Applying the beam to the full circumference of the ureteral wall leads to stricture formation. This is indicated only if the goal is to occlude

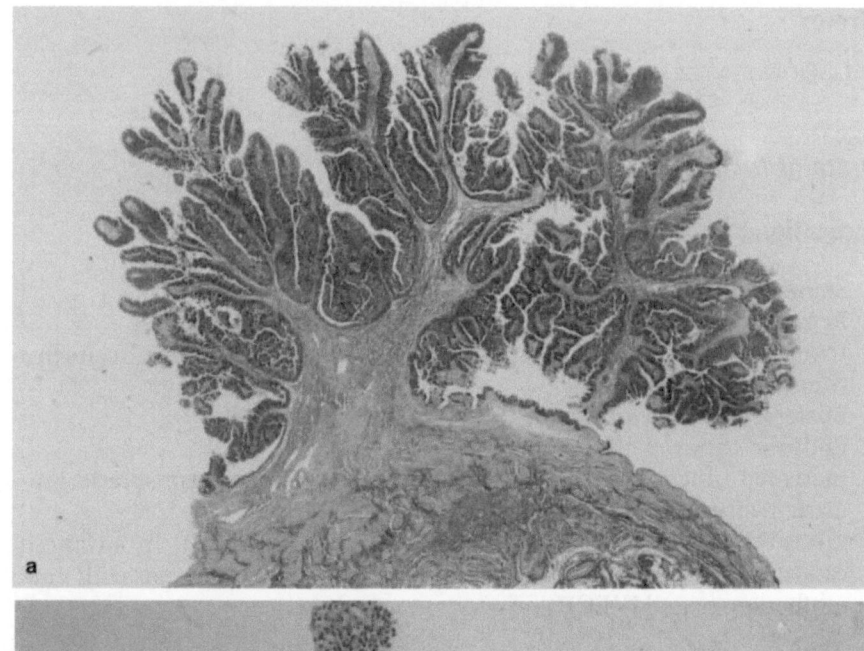

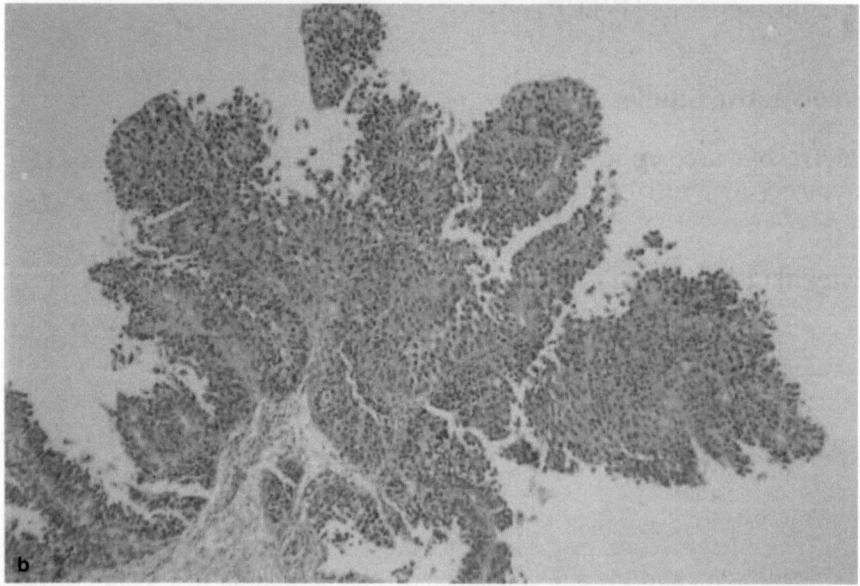

Fig. 4.28. a Papillary ureteral tumor–histological appearance before laser treatment (van Gieson stain). **b** After laser treatment, the tumor exhibits the same basic histological pattern. H&E stain

Fig. 4.29. Tumor location
at ureteroscopy (schematic
view)

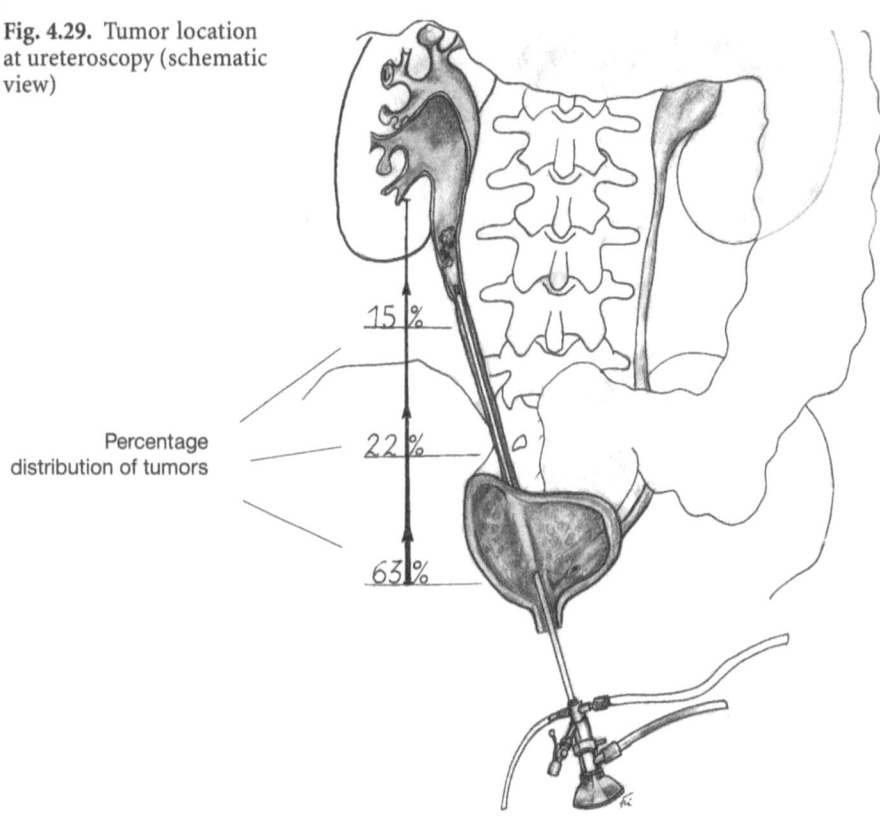

Percentage
distribution of tumors

15 %

22 %

63 %

the ureter of a nephrostomized kidney, in which case an antegrade technique is used, i.e., the laser fiber is advanced to the desired level of the ureter through the nephrostomy, and the ureter is circumferentially lased at a power output of 30 W.

Advantage

- Organ preservation

Disadvantage

- Need for regular follow-up examinations

Fig. 4.30. *Single* laser pulses (20–30 W) are applied for selective destruction of the tumor base

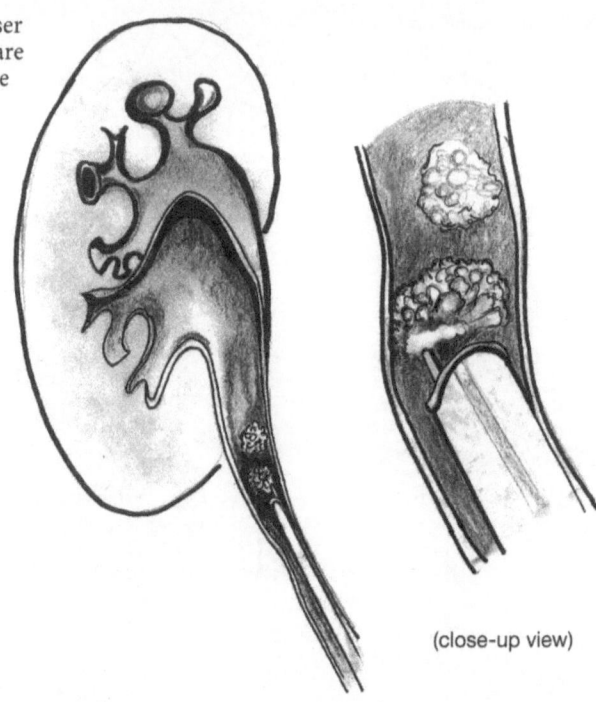

(close-up view)

Fig. 4.31. The lased tumor is removed with rigid or flexible biopsy forceps

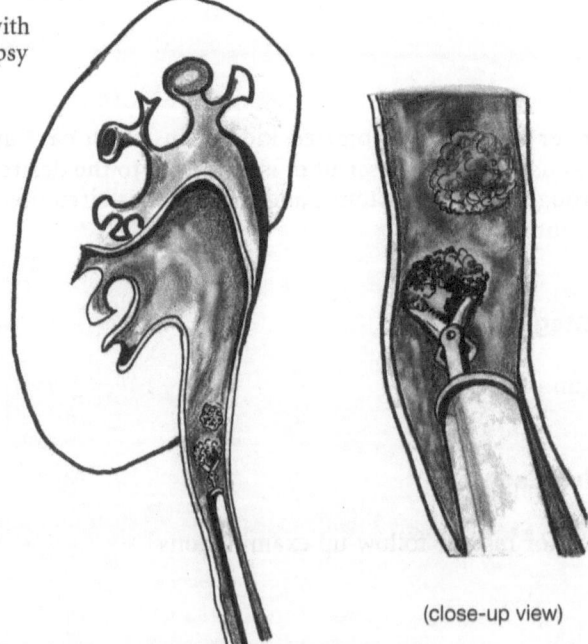

(close-up view)

Fig. 4.32. The laser is reapplied to the tumor bed

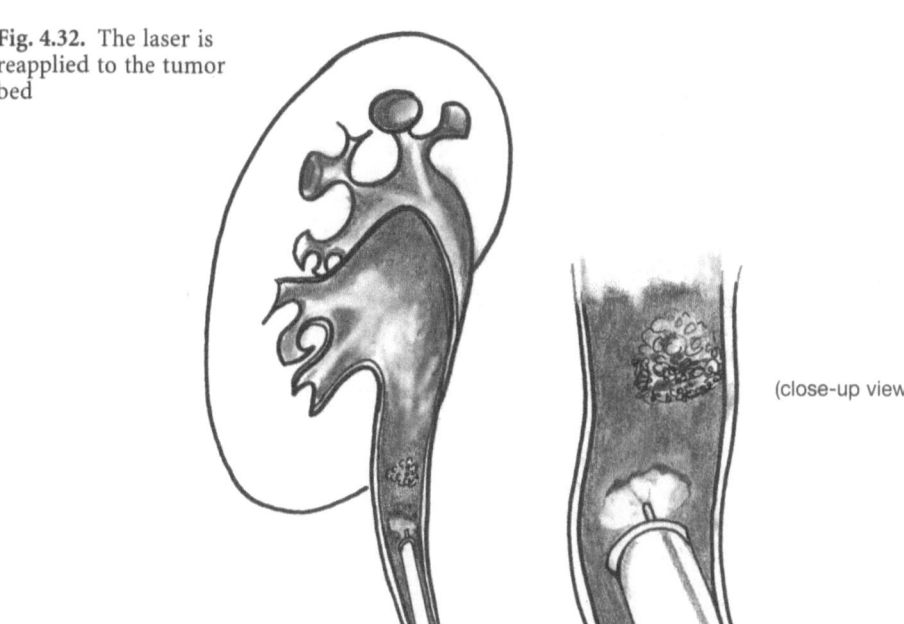

(close-up view)

Follow-up

- During the first year after tumor removal:
  - Every 3 months: ureteroscopy, biopsy, cytology, and ultrasound
  - Every 6 months: CT, bone scan, bone marrow biopsy
- During the second year:
  - Every 6 months: ureteroscopy, biopsy, cytology, and ultrasound
  - Adjunctive studies: CT, bone scan, bone marrow biopsy
- After two years:
  - Every 9 months: ureteroscopy, biopsy, cytology, and ultrasound
  - Adjunctive studies: CT, bone scan, bone marrow biopsy
- After four years:
  - Annual ureteroscopy, biopsy, cytology, and ultrasound
  - Adjunctive studies: CT, bone scan, bone marrow biopsy
  - Recurrent tumor is managed and followed in the same way as a primary tumor.

Contraindications

- Multiple tumors widely involving the ureter and poorly differentiated tumors (grade III).

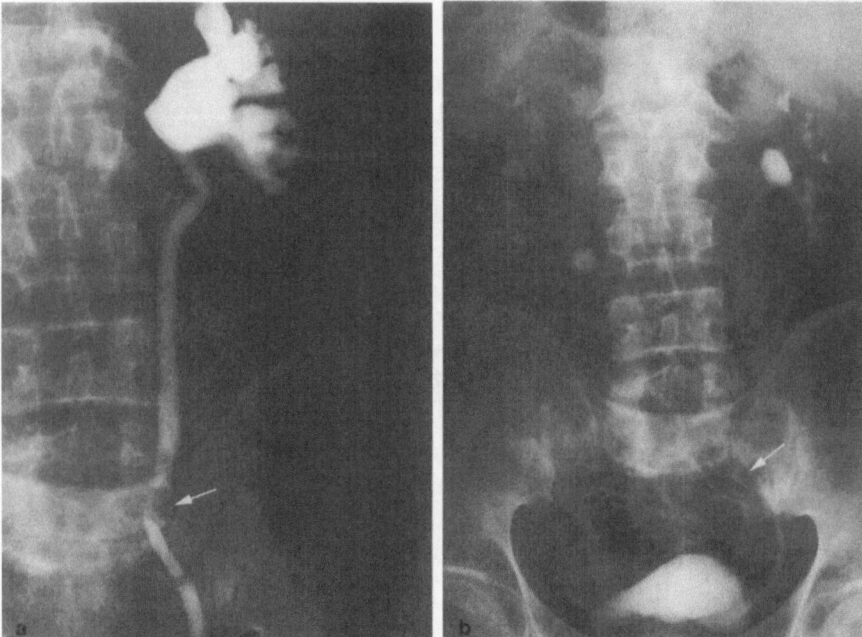

Fig. 4.33. a Urogram preceding the laser treatment of a ureteral tumor. **b** Urogram following laser treatment of a ureteral tumor (*arrow*)

- Also: the same contraindications that are observed in patients with bladder cancer (see Sect. 4.3.1).

Instrumentation

- Rigid ureterorenoscope (Ch 7.5–11.0).
- Flexible ureterorenoscope (Ch 6–12.0).

4.5
Pyelocaliceal System

A.G. HOFSTETTER

4.5.1
Pyelocaliceal Tumors

Indications

- Same as for ureteral tumors (see Sect. 4.4.1).

Preoperative Studies

- Intravenous urography/lavage cytology, ureteropyeloscopy, and biopsies.

Screening for Metastases

- CT, bone scan, bone marrow biopsy, chest radiographs

Operative Technique

- Routes of approach:
  - Open exposure of the kidney with pyelocalicotomy or nephrotomy. If necessary, partial nephrectomy is performed using crushed ice to cool the kidney (Fig. 4.34).
  - Ureteropelviscopy (see Sect. 4.4.1) and nephroscopy (Fig. 4.35).
  - Pyelocaliceal nephroscopy (Fig. 4.35).

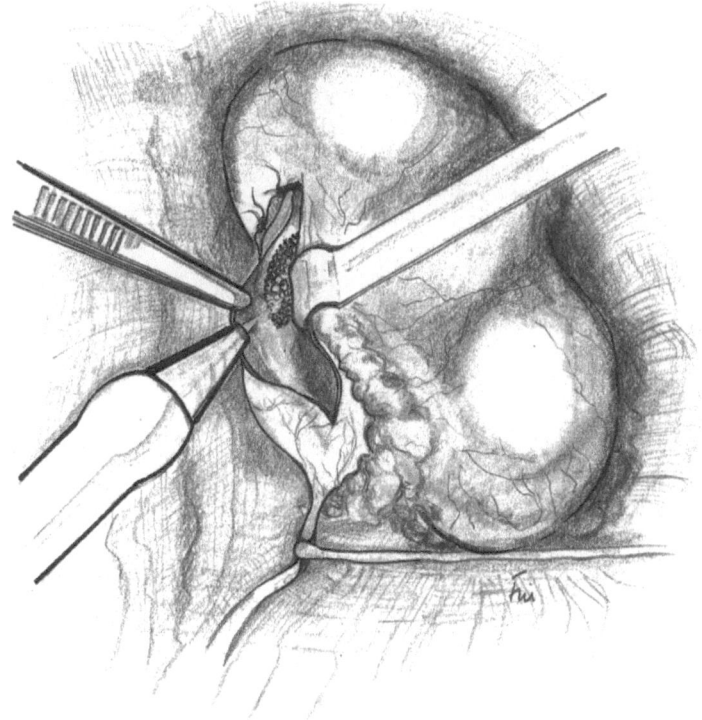

Fig. 4.34. Renal pelvic tumors are exposed by a pyelocalicotomy and coagulated with a defocused Nd:YAG laser beam (20 W)

Fig. 4.35a–c. Possible approaches for laser surgery of the pyelocaliceal system.
a Ureteroscopic approach.
b Nephroscopic access to the upper and lower caliceal groups. **c** Nephroscopic access to the middle caliceal group

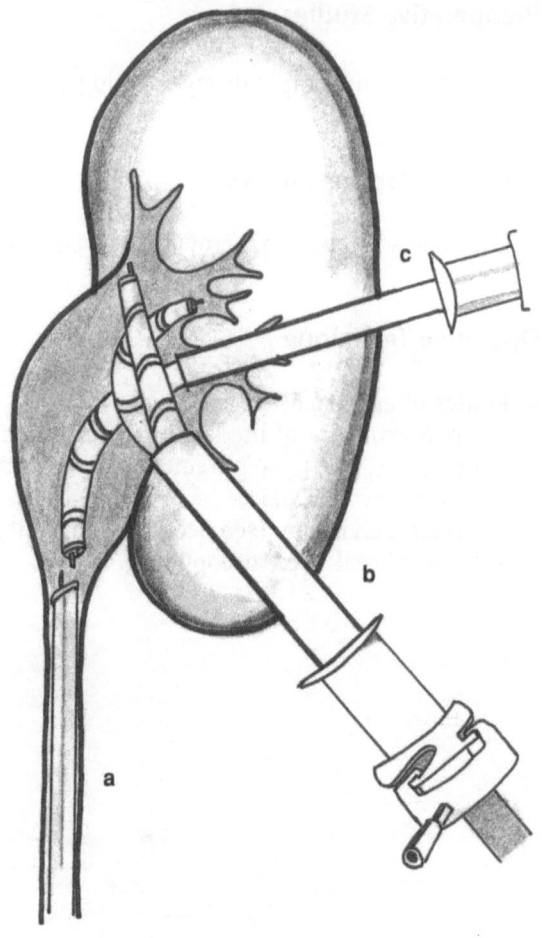

Technique

- Open exposure of the kidney through an intercostal incision affords the best view.
- A pyelotomy, pyelocalicotomy, nephrotomy, or partial nephrectomy (with or without crushed-ice hypothermia) may be performed, depending on the location of the tumor and anatomic conditions.
- After the tumor has been exposed, it is lased at a distance of 4–8 mm using a focused or defocused beam at 30–35 W until the tissue whitens.
- The necrotic tumor is removed with biopsy forceps, and the material is submitted for pathology.
- After the exophytic portion of the tumor has been removed, the laser is reapplied to coagulate the tumor bed.

Instrumentation

- Teflon-coated quartz fiber with a special handpiece, protective eyewear.
- If the percutaneous approach is used (Fig. 4.35), access to the tumor is established through a pyelocaliceal nephrostomy. The laser quartz fiber is directed to the tumor site through a Ch 24 or 26 nephroscope (rigid or flexible), with or without an Albarran deflector, while continuous water irrigation is maintained. Various viewing telescopes (0°, 30°, 70°) are used (Fig. 4.36).
- Distance of laser fiber from tumor: 1–2 mm. The power delivered to the tissue should not exceed 30 W.
- The laser beam is applied in linear passes until the tumor tissue has whitened.
- The exophytic portion of the mass is removed with biopsy forceps, and the tumor bed is coagulated at 30 W.

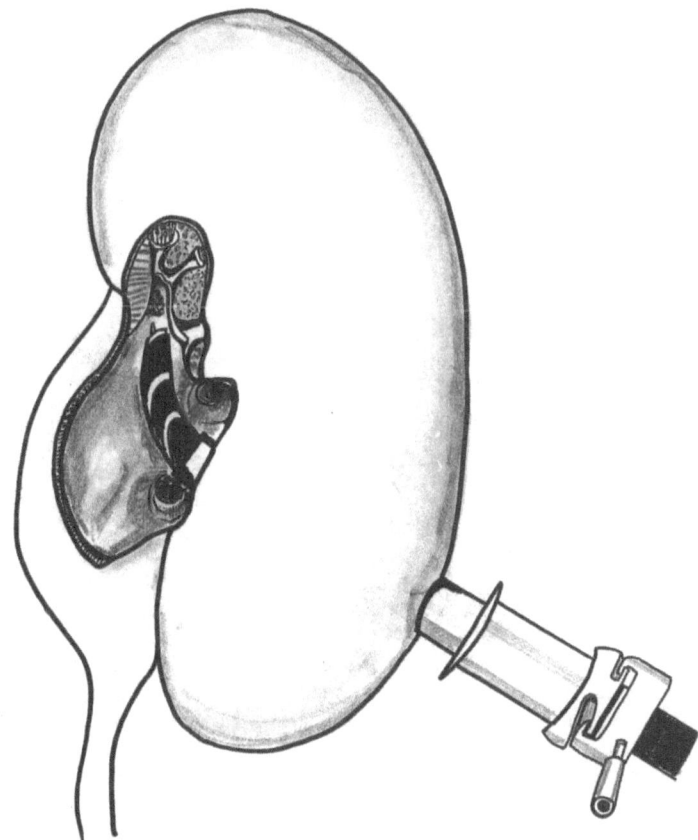

Fig. 4.36. A flexible nephroscope is introduced through a pyelocaliceal nephrostomy for the laser destruction of a small caliceal tumor (power output: 20 W)

Ureteropelviscopic tumor destruction follows the same basic technique as the ureteroscopic treatment of ureteral tumors (Fig. 4.35a).

Advantages and Disadvantages

- Same as for ureteral tumors (see Sect. 4.4.1)

Follow-up

- Same as for ureteral tumors (see Sect. 4.4.1)

Contraindications

- Small hydronephrotic kidney.
- The same contraindications that apply to ureteral tumors (see Sect. 4.4.1).

Instrumentation

- Nephroscope (Ch 24–26)
- Assorted endoscopes (0°, 30°, and 70°)

References

Friesen A, Schilling A, Keiditsch E (1987) Untersuchungen zur Laserchirurgie am Harnleiter. Verh Dtsch Ges Urol 38:386–387

Hofstetter AG (1988) Laserkoagulationsbehandlung von Urotheltumoren im oberen Harntrakt. In: Schuler J, Hofstetter AG (eds) Endourologie. Thieme, Stuttgart, pp 158–164

Hofstetter AG, Frank F (1979) Der Nd:YAG-Laser in der Urologie. Roche, Basel

Hofstetter AG, Keiditsch E (1985) Lasers for renal pelvic and ureteral tumors. Laser I:75–78

Hofstetter AG, Bowering G, Keiditsch E, Frank F (1983) Zerstörung von Uretertumoren mit dem Nd-YAG-Laser – ein neues, organerhaltendes Operationsverfahren. Fortschr Med 101:625–627

Malloy TR (1985) Laser treatment of ureter and upper collecting system. In: Lasers in urological surgery. Smith JA (ed) Year Book Medical, Chicago, pp 82–93

Pensel J, Schmeller N, Unsold T, Kriegmair M, Hofstetter AG (1986) Percutaneous ureter occlusion with Nd-YAG-Laser. In: Waidelich W, Kiefhaber P (1986) Laser/Opto-elektronik in der Medizin. Springer, Berlin Heidelberg New York, pp 530–531

Rassweiler JF, Eisenberger F (1986) Tumoren der Urogenitalorgane. In: Hofstetter AG, Eisenberger G (eds) Urologie für die Praxis. Bergmann, Munich

Schmeller N, Hofstetter AG (1989) Laser treatment of ureteral tumors. J Urol 141:840–843

Smith JA (1983) Nd:YAG laser photoirradiation of canine ureters. Surg Forum 34:696–697

4.6
Laparoscopic Pelvic Lymphadenectomy

W. LUBOS, N. SCHMELLER, and A.G. HOFSTETTER

In the treatment of prostatic cancer that appears to be localized, there has been a growing trend in recent years to tailor the treatment to the stage of the disease (Austenfeld and Bradley 1990). The pelvic lymph node status is a particularly important criterion. Finding even a single regional micrometastasis implies a significantly poorer prognosis in terms of tumor progression and likelihood of survival (Gervasi et al. 1989) and calls for a differentiated therapeutic approach. While radical prostatovesiculectomy is the preferred treatment for patients without lymph node metastases (Walsh et al. 1992), positive lymph nodes are an indication for systemic therapy in the form of androgen deprivation using surgical (plastic orchiectomy) or pharmacological means (e.g., antiandrogens).

As there is no published proof that multimodal therapy (radical prostatovesiculectomy plus androgen deprivation) is more effective than androgen deprivation alone in patients with positive nodes, it would be beneficial to ascertain the patient's lymph node status without resorting to open surgery. Because imaging procedures (ultrasound, CT, MRI, lymphangiography) have proven too imprecise for evaluating the pelvic lymph nodes, laparoscopic pelvic lymphadenectomy, first described by Schuessler et al (1991), is the only procedure at present that satisfies the requirements of accuracy and low invasiveness.

In bladder cancer as in cancer of the prostate, involvement of the pelvic lymph nodes marks the transition from localized to systemic disease. Since CT, MRI, and ultrasound cannot guarantee accurate pelvic lymph node staging, laparoscopic pelvic lymphadenectomy is again of critical importance as a prelude to radical cystectomy (Skinner et al. 1991; Smith and Whitmore 1991).

Indications

- Histologically confirmed prostate cancer (GI and/or PSA no less than 10 mg/ml) or bladder cancer, or to exclude lymph node involvement before a planned prostatovesiculectomy or cystectomy.

Preoperative Studies

- Operability and age: laparoscopic pelvic lymphadenectomy is appropriate only if the *age* and *constitution* of the patient would permit a radical prostatectomy or curative radiotherapy to be performed if a negative lymph node status is confirmed.
- Clinical tumor stage: Ta–T4 (Walsh et al. 1992), Nx, M0.

Screening for Metastases

Mandatory screening studies include CT, MRI, lymph node biopsy if required, biplane chest radiographs, and bone scans.

The workup of prostatic carcinoma should always include a serum assay of prostate-specific antigen (PSA). The serum PSA level can provide evidence of lymph node metastases. In a study by Oesterling et al (1988), approximately 75 % of 20 patients with a serum PSA higher than 20 ng/ml were found to have involvement of lymph nodes or the seminal vesicles.

Operative Technique

Preoperative Preparations

- All patients selected for a laparoscopic lymphadenectomy must undergo a thorough physical examination. The presumption of significant bowel adhesions may contraindicate the procedure in patients who have had previous lower abdominal surgery.
- The patient is informed about the possible need for open surgery, and informed consent is obtained.
- There is no need for routine antegrade intestinal lavage or the preoperative administration of a broad-spectrum antibiotic. The bowel should be well evacuated, however, since distention of the sigmoid colon by gas or stool would obstruct the surgeon's view. Preoperative low-dose heparinization is usually given.

Operative Method

General endotracheal anesthesia is administered to ensure total relaxation. All standard instruments for abdominal surgery are laid out along with the laparoscopic instruments. A video cart with a monitor (e.g., CCD Endocam 5370 with Endocolor system) is placed at the foot of the operating table. A high-intensity light source and CO_2 insufflator are positioned to one side, opposite the surgeon (Fig. 4.37).

The camera-holding assistant is also stationed opposite the surgeon. The bladder is routinely catheterized to keep the bladder empty during the procedure. First the patient is placed in the Trendelenburg position, and the Veress needle with valve open is inserted through the umbilical fossa while the abdominal wall is pulled upward. An aspiration test is performed after the instillation of 20 ml NaCl to confirm correct needle placement.

A pneumoperitoneum is then established by insufflating CO_2 through the Veress needle to a maximum pressure of 14 mmHg. The gas flow for initial insufflation is limited to 1 l/min. The pneumoperitoneum is now probed with a 0.8-mm cannula, and gas is aspirated at the proposed site of trocar

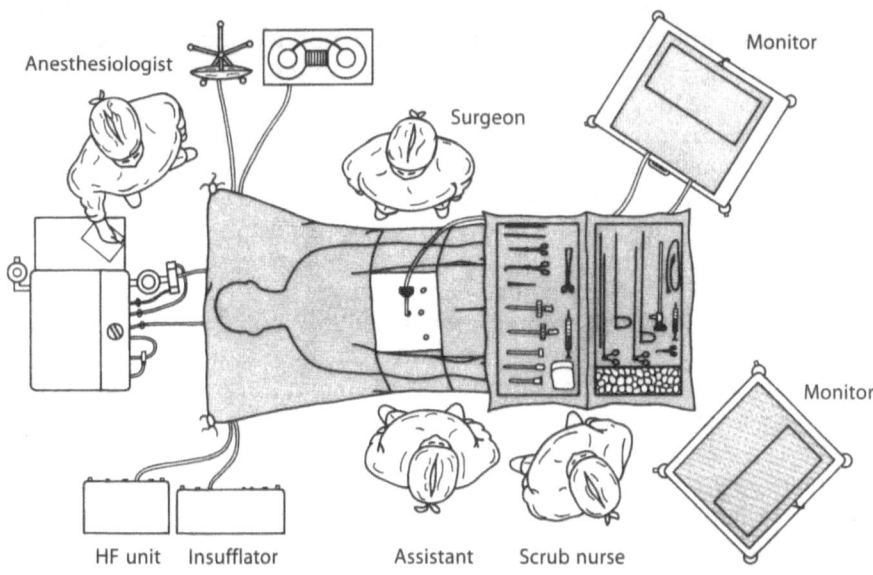

Fig. 4.37. Suggested arrangement of operating room personnel, equipment, and port sites for laparoscopic pelvic lymphadenectomy

Fig. 4.38. Placement of ports for laparoscopic pelvic lymphade-nectomy

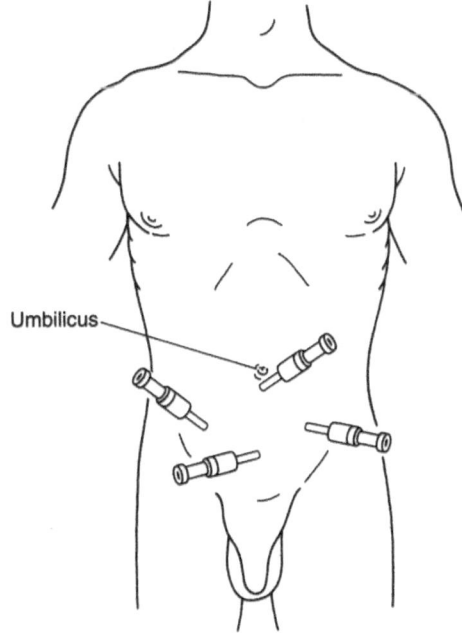

insertion. Following the blind, transumbilical insertion of the 11-mm primary trocar through a Z incision using the Semm technique (Fig. 4.38), the videoendoscope is introduced and connected to the CO_2 insufflator tubing. When inserting the trocar, the surgeon should hold the extended index finger firmly against the sheath to keep the trocar from plunging too deeply when it surmounts the resistance of the abdominal wall. In thin patients, the aortic bifurcation often lies only 10 cm behind the umbilicus.

With the videoendoscope in the abdomen, a pair of 5-mm trocars are inserted two fingerwidths medial to the left and right anterior superior iliac spines under direct vision, and a 5- or 10-mm trocar is inserted on the midline between the umbilicus and symphysis or at a pararectal site that is level with the umbilicus. The second 10-mm trocar provides access for the clip-applying forceps. It is even better to use an 11-mm trocar, for when the CO_2 insufflation tubing is connected, the gap between the 10-mm instrument and the 11-mm sheath permits a much higher rate of gas inflow. Cold gas from the compression tank entering the telescope sheath causes rapid fogging of the lens system and can seriously hamper visibility.

With experience, we have found that an instrument passed through a 10- or 11-mm midline port often interferes with the telescope, so we prefer to locate this port at a pararectal site midway between the 5-mm working port and the umbilicus, at a level slightly below the umbilicus. The zone of the epigastric artery, extending medially from the McBurney point to the rectus above the symphysis pubis, should be strictly avoided due to the risk of hemorrhage.

The ports having been established, the patient is placed in a laterally rotated Trendelenburg position to help displace bowel loops from the side that is to be inspected. The surgeon may have to free sigmoid colon adhesions to obtain a clear view of the area of the lymph node dissection. This area lies distal to the common iliac bifurcation, lateral to the medial umbilical ligament (the usually obliterated umbilical artery), medial to the external iliac artery and genitofemoral nerve, and superior to the os pubis (Fig. 4.39).

The posterior peritoneal membrane is initially opened along the external iliac artery over the superior pubic ramus, lateral to the umbilical ligament, carrying the incision toward the hypogastric artery to the bifurcation of the common iliac artery. If visibility of the operative site is restricted, the vas deferens should be doubly clipped and divided with the laser Fibertome. If a total lymphadenectomy is planned, the obturator nerve is exposed from its site of entry into the obturator canal to its crossing of the iliac vein.

Then the lymph node chains are dissected free, coagulated with the laser Fibertome, and resected inferiorly at the level of the superior pubic ramus (Fig. 4.40). If possible, the tissue is removed en bloc with a 10-mm extractor passed through the 11-mm working channel. Lymph nodes too large to pass through the working channel can be fragmented in an entrapment sack for frozen-section evaluation or removed through a 15-mm trocar, or a Tru-cut biopsy or partial resection of the suspicious lymph node can be performed if the node is fixed. If frozen sections confirm lymph node metastasis, the contralateral lymph nodes are left alone.

The procedure concludes with meticulous hemostasis, irrigation of the wound and cul-de-sac, desufflation of the abdomen, and removal of the trocars under vision. Generally there is no need to insert drains.

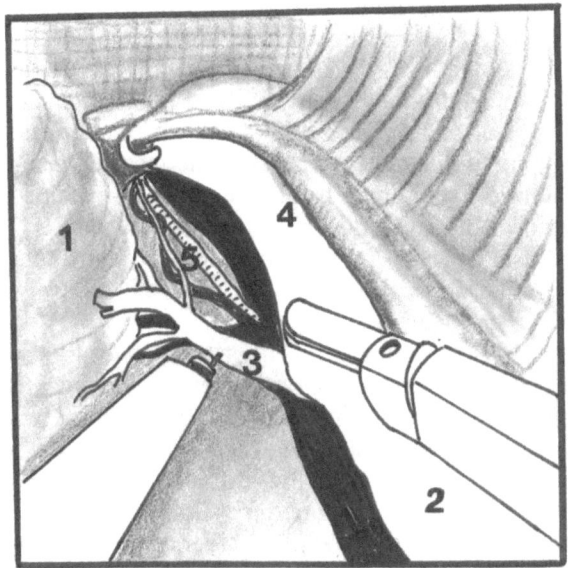

Fig. 4.39. Schematic view of the lymphadenectomy region. *1*, Bladder; *2*, common iliac artery; *3*, internal iliac artery, *4*, external iliac artery; *5*, obturator fossa containing the obturator artery and vein and the obturator nerve

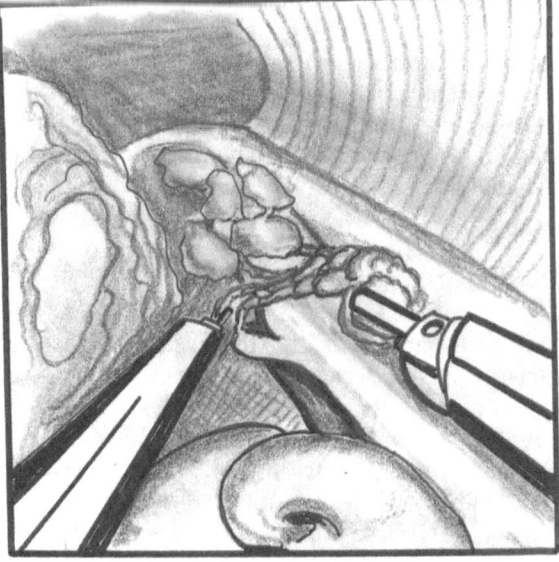

Fig. 4.40. Appearance of the field during a laparoscopic lymphadenectomy. Dissection and coagulation of the nodal package with the Nd:YAG laser prevents the complication of lymphorrhea

Advantages over Conventional Methods

A major advantage is the lower complication rate compared with conventional open lymphadenectomy. Complications occurred in 19 % of 69 patients who underwent laparoscopic surgery, and their complications were consistently milder than in a comparison group that had open surgery ($n=59$). The latter group had almost twice the complication rate, at 37 %, and two patients developed serious complications (sepsis and pneumonia). The most frequent complication following pelvic lymphadenectomy was obstructed lymphatic drainage with lymphocele formation. While laparoscopic lymphadenectomy with the laser Fibertome could not prevent lymphocele formation, the incidence of this complication, at 5 %, was lower than in the conventional laparoscopy group (8.7 %) and open surgery patients (13.6 %). As an added benefit, the laparoscopic window provides minimally invasive access for treating this frequent complication (McCollough et al. 1991).

Superior hemostasis. The average blood loss in 69 patients was 270 ml. The laser Fibertome proved very advantageous in this regard, reducing blood loss by an average of 90 ml compared with conventional high-frequency monopolar electrocautery. This can be attributed to the shorter coagulation time with the laser Fibertome and the more rapid sealing of blood vessels, creating better visibility for the surgeon. The laser Fibertome also appears to reduce the incidence of lymphocele formation.

Less cardiovascular stress owing to a reduction in surgical trauma. Wound pain is diminished, and most patients can get out of bed on the first postoperative day. Cosmetic acceptability is another advantage of laparoscopic lymphadenectomy over open surgery.

Because definitive treatment – radical prostatectomy, cystectomy, or androgen ablation therapy – is performed in a later session, the patient has time to decide on a therapeutic option based on the evaluation of his lymph node status. Also, the staged nature of the therapy avoids the risks of overtreatment or inadequate treatment resulting from a high rate of false-negative frozen sections (Steinberg et al. 1990).

Disadvantages

One disadvantage is the relatively long procedure time, which averaged 166 min in our series but improved with practice: the first ten operations lasted an average of 207 min, the last 10 only 140 min. Laser-assisted laparoscopic pelvic lymphadenectomy places increased technical demands on the surgeon, who must master proper laser technique in addition to standard laparoscopic techniques.

Comprehensive equipment is needed both for the laser surgery and for the eventuality of converting to open laparotomy. One cost-saving factor is the smaller surgical team; generally only one assistant is needed instead of the two or three required for open lymphadenectomy.

There is a theoretical but unsubstantiated risk of seeding tumor cells into the abdominal cavity during a Tru-cut biopsy or partial lymphadenectomy. This risk can perhaps be eliminated by using a special entrapment sack for tissue retrieval such as that described by Kavoussi and Clayman (1992). In the clinical series described here, we found that the handling of the sack was cumbersome. Also, the issue of tumor cell spillage may have no clinical relevance given the fact that, once lymphogenous spread has occurred, the patient has a systemic disease that is no longer amenable to local treatment.

Follow-up

Follow-ups are not scheduled for patients who have been selected for a second operation (radical prostatectomy). If lower abdominal complaints arise (lymphocele formation!), the patient should be evaluated by ultrasound and intravenous urography or cystourethrography.

Contraindication

• Confirmed metastasis

Instrumentation

Basically the same instruments are used for laparoscopic pelvic lymphadenectomy as for general laparoscopic surgery. The laser Fibertome (Medilas 4060 N) is used in the "Fibertome mode" in which a feedback circuit automatically adjusts the power output in response to tissue effect. When the laser is first activated, the maximum photoradiation setting should be selected (1–3 in the Fibertome mode). At this setting an algorithm adjusts the laser power output to match the preset tissue temperature.

References

Austenfeld MS, Bradley ED (1990) New concepts in the treatment of stage D1 adeno-carcinoma of the prostate. Urol Clin North Am 17:867

Castellino RA, Ray G, Blank N, Govan D, Bagshaw M (1973) Lymphangiograpy in prostatic carcinoma: preliminary observations. JAMA 223:877

Gervasi LA, Mata J, Easley JD, Wilbanks JH, Seale-Hawkins C, Carlton CE Jr, Scardino PT (1989) Prognostic significance of lymph nodal metastasis in prostate cancer. J Urol 142:332

Kavoussi LR, Claymann RV (1992) Organ entrapment system for removing nodal tissue during laparoscopic pelvic lymphadenectomy. J Urol 147:879

Lee JK, Stanley RJ, Sagel SS, McClennan BL (1978) Accuracy of CT in detecting intraabdominal and pelvic lymph node metastases from pelvic cancers. J Roentgen 131:675

McCollough CS, Soper NJ, Clayman RV (1991) Laparoscopic drainage of a posttransplant lymphocele. Transplantation 51:725

Oesterling JE, Chan DW, Epstein JI et al (1988) Prostate specific antigen in the preoperative and postoperative evaluation of localized prostate cancer treated with radical prostatectomy. J Urol 139:766

Pagano F et al (1991) Results of contemporary radical cystectomy for invasive bladder cancer: a clinicopathological study with an emphasis on the inadequacy of the tumor, nodes and metastasis classification. J Urol 146:45

Parra PO, Andrus C, Boullier J (1992) Staging laparoscopic pelvic lymph node dissection: comparison of results with open pelvic lymphadenectomy. J Urol 147:857

Rifkin MD, Zerhouni EA, Gatsonis CA, Quint LE, Paushter DM et al (1990) Comparison of magnetic resonance imaging and ultrasonography in staging early prostate cancer. N Engl J Med 323:621

Roehrborn CAJ, Sagalowsky PC et al (1991) Long-term patient survival for regional metastatic transitional cell carcinoma of the bladder. J Urol 146:36

Schmeller N, Lubos W, Theodorakis J, Fabricius P-G (1993) Laparoskopische pelvine Lymphadenektomie. MMW 135:193

Schuessler WW, Vancaille TG, Reich H, Griffith DP (1991) Transperitoneal endosurgical lymphhadenectomy in patients with localized prostate cancer. J Urol 145:988

Skinner DG et al (1991) The role of adjuvant chemotherapy following cystectomy for invasive bladder cancer: a prospective comparative trial. J Urol 145:459

Smith JA, Whitmore WF (1981) Regional lymph node metastasis from bladder cancer. J Urol 126:591

Splinter TAW et al (1992) The prognostic value of the pathological response to combination chemotherapy before cystectomy in patients with invasive bladder cancer. J Urol 147:606

Steinberg GD, Epstein JI, Pintadose S, Walsh PC (1990) Management of stage D1 adenocarcinoma of the prostate: The Johns Hopkins experience 1974 to 1987. J Urol 144:1425

Walsh PC, Retik AB, Stamey TA, Vaughan ED (1992) Campbell's Urology. Saunders, Philadelphia pp 1209–1214

Winfield HN, Donovan JF, See WA, Loening SA, Williams RD (1992) Laparoscopic pelvic lymph node dissection for genitourinary malignancies: indications, techniques and results. J Endourol 6:103

4.7
Laser-Assisted Vasovasostomy

A. FRIESEN

As vasectomy becomes increasing popular as a contraceptive method, growing numbers of patients are presenting with a desire for vasectomy reversal. Conventional vasovasostomy is performed under the operating microscope using a two-layered anastomotic suture technique.

Building on the knowledge gained from laser-assisted vascular anastomoses (Jarrow et al. 1986), researchers in the early 1980s began to report initial experience with laser-assisted vasovasostomy (LAVVS) in laboratory animals (Lynne et al. 1983). The procedure was first performed in patients in 1986 (Rosenberg 1987; Rosenberg et al. 1985, 1988).

The goal of laser-assisted vasovasostomy is to provide a simple technique that facilitates the difficult procedure of microsurgical vasovasostomy.

Experimental vasovasostomy with the CO_2 laser (Alefeld et al. 1991; Seidmann et al. 1990) produced success rates equivalent to those of conventional therapy, despite the fact that tissue penetration was limited to the serosa and adjacent portions of the muscularis. Lasers of other wavelengths have been tried in an effort to eliminate intramural sperm granulomas, but so far the Nd:YAG laser, with its deeper tissue penetration, has produced inconsistent results no better than those obtained with the CO_2 laser.

Clinical application in small numbers of patients confirms a patency rate equivalent to that of conventional surgery (Shanberg et al. 1990).

Indication

- Azoospermia following vasectomy

Operative Technique

- The scrotal contents are exposed through a scrotal or inguinal incision. The vas deferens is exposed, preserving its blood supply, and the vasectomy scar is identified.
- The vas deferens is sharply divided on both sides. Aspirate from the distal portion of the vas is microscopically evaluated, and the patency of the proximal segment is tested.
- The vasal stumps are approximated using two or more 9-0 or 10-0 all-layer coapting sutures (Fig. 4.41). Successful laser welding requires absolute dryness at the anastomotic site. The seromuscular anastomosis is performed by CO_2 laser photocoagulation of the area between the sutures.
- The laser power output is 90-120 mW with a spot size of 0.1 mm and a pulse duration of 0.1 s.

Fig. 4.41. Laser-assisted vasovasostomy. The transsected vasa are reapproximated with full-thickness 10-0 interrupted sutures in preparation for laser welding

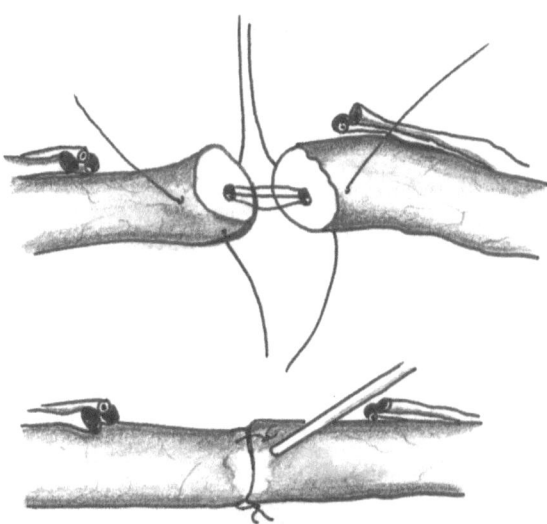

Advantages over Conventional Technique

- Laser welding simplifies an otherwise tedious and more technically demanding operation.
- Laser welding shortens the operative time.
- The use of fewer coapting sutures reduces surgical trauma.

Disadvantages

- High equipment costs.

Patient numbers are still too small to document any superiority of laser-assisted vasovasostomy over microsurgical technique. Research in this area is continuing.

References

Alefelder J et al (1991) Stented laser-welded vasovasostomy in the rat: comparison of Nd:YAG and CO$_2$ lasers. J Reconstr Microsurg 7:317–320

Jarrow J, Cooley B, Marshall FF (1986) Laser-assisted vasal anastomosis in the rat and man. J Urol 36:1132–1135

Lynne CM et al (1983) Laser-assisted vas anastomosis. A preliminary report. Lasers Surg Med 3:260–263

Rosenberg SK (1987) Clinical use of carbon dioxide (CO$_2$) laser in microsurgical vasovasostomy. Urol 29:372–374

Rosenberg SK et al (1985) Carbon dioxide (CO$_2$) laser in microsurgical vasovasostomy. Urology 25:53–56

Rosenberg SK et al (1988) Further clinical experience with (CO$_2$) laser in microsurgical vasovasostomy. Urology 32:225–227

Seidmann EL et al (1990) Vasovasostomy in dogs using the carbon dioxide milliwatt laser. II. Lasers Surg Med 10:433–437

Shanberg A et al (1990) Laser-assisted vasectomy reversal: experience in 32 patients. J Urol 143:528–530

4.8
Prostate

R. Muschter and A.G. Hofstetter

By the late 1970 s there were already published reports on initial experience with the Nd:YAG laser in the treatment of prostatic diseases (Böwering et al. 1979; Camey and Le Duc 1980). In the years that followed, several groups of authors focused on the treatment of prostatic carcinoma (Beisland 1990; McNicholas et al. 1988; Sander and Beisland 1984; Vahlensieck et al. 1990). Broad clinical application followed several years later, marked by the parallel development of various therapeutic techniques (Costello et al. 1992a,b; Hofstetter 1991; Johnson et al. 1991; Muschter et al. 1992a; Roth and Aretz

1991). Today lasers are used in the treatment of benign and malignant prostatic tumors that are associated with bladder outlet obstruction. The curative treatment of prostate cancer is still experimental in nature.

4.8.1
Benign Prostatic Hyperplasia

The goal of the laser treatment of benign prostatic hyperplasia (BPH) is to relieve bladder outlet obstruction and other symptoms. In most techniques this is carried out by the direct or secondary ablation of tissue. Available techniques consist of transurethral contact incision and resection, transurethral contact and noncontact vaporization, and transurethral and interstitial coagulation of the prostate. These techniques are also practiced in various combinations.

The nomenclature of laser treatments for BPH is:

- Transurethral incision of the prostate (TUIP)
- Transurethral ultrasound-guided laser-induced prostatectomy (TULIP)
- Visual/endoscopic laser ablation of the prostate (VLAP, ELAP, LAP)
- Interstitial laser coagulation/thermotherapy (ILC, LITT, ITT)
- Transurethral laser ablation/vaporization of the prostate (TULAP)
- Contact laser vaporization
- Transurethral balloon laser prostatectomy
- Holmium laser ablation of the prostate (HoLAP)
- Combined endoscopic laser ablation of the prostate (CELAP)
- Holmium laser resection of the prostate (HoLRP)

Indications

- All techniques have basically the same indications: Vahlensieck stage II, III or IV disease with significant obstructive symptoms.

Preoperative Studies

The preoperative workup includes the history, general clinical and urological examinations, and special neurological studies. A florid infection involving the urinary tract or seminiferous structures must be excluded or treated.

Specific studies: determination of the International Prostatic Symptom Score (IPSS) and quality of life index, uroflowmetry, ultrasound determination of residual urine, and transrectal ultrasound. Urodynamic evaluation is not performed routinely but is a helpful study and should be performed if possible.

Since the laser treatment of BPH does not provide material for histological evaluation, the presence of prostate cancer must be excluded (DRE, PSA, TRUS, biopsy if necessary).

Operative Technique

Transurethral Laser Incision of the Prostate

This procedure is best suited for small adenomas, also for isolated, relatively small median lobes and adenomatous lesions that involve a high transverse bar (Shanberg et al. 1985).

Transurethral incision of the prostate can be performed with the Nd:YAG laser, but a holmium:YAG or KTP laser can also be used. The incision can be made by contact with a bare fiber or by placing a delivery system designed for noncontact use in direct contact with the tissue. Special contact tips are also available in various shapes and designs.

The light guide is advanced into the bladder through a urethrocystoscope, placed in contact with the prostate at the bladder neck, and slowly withdrawn to the seminal colliculus while continuous laser energy is applied. Several such passes are made in the same position, gradually deepening the incision to the level of the trigone. In principle, any number of incisions can be made at any position, but generally the incision is made either at 6 o'clock or at 5 and 7 o'clock (lithotomy position). If a contact tip is used, the incision can be performed in the reverse direction, i.e., by moving the fiber inward from the prostatic apex toward the bladder neck.

The power output is 20–60 W. The Fibertome is used at setting 2 with an output of 40–60 W.

Transurethral Laser Resection of the Prostate

The immediate goal of this technique, as in transurethral electroresection of the prostate (TURP), is the excision of prostatic tissue. Reportedly, LRP is associated with lighter and less frequent bleeding than TURP (Gilling et al. 1995, 1996). The resection is the result of multiple incisions, which may be arranged in a wedge-shaped pattern (as in the Nesbit technique of transurethral prostatectomy).

We use a holmium laser for the resection, but an Nd:YAG laser or diode laser would probably be suitable as well. As with simple incision of the prostate, the resection is performed with a bare fiber placed in direct contact with the tissue. An Nd:YAG or diode laser can be used with a bare fiber or with a contact tip.

The light guide is advanced into the bladder through a urethrocystoscope and placed in contact with the prostate at the bladder neck. Then the fiber is drawn slowly outward toward the apex while continuous laser energy is applied. Multiple passes are made in the same position, deepening the incision until it reaches the capsule. The next series of passes is made in a different position, still directing the beam toward the same area of the capsule. This results in the excision of a large, wedge-shaped piece of prostatic tissue, which initially is pushed into the bladder.

As an alternative, the second incision may be carried along the plane of the capsule to form the base of the wedge. The resection starts anteriorly and proceeds inwards to the next wedge until all of the lobe has been removed. If the prostate is very long, it can be divided in half at the midgland level, and the basal portions can be resected first, followed by the apical portions (much as in a conventional TURP). When the resection has been completed, the tissue fragments are flushed out of the bladder. Larger pieces should be morcellated while still in the urethra or inside the bladder if necessary before they are removed.

The pulsed Ho:YAG laser delivers a continuous power output of 60 W with a pulse energy of 2.4 J and a repetition rate of 25 Hz. A power output of 60 W or more is recommended for laser resections of the prostate to ensure a high cutting rate and effective hemostasis (although a lower mean output can also produce an acceptable cutting effect). For the same reasons, the Nd:YAG or diode laser should be operated at 40–100 W. The Fibertome should be operated at a setting of 2 or 3 with a power output of 40–100 W.

Transurethral Contact Laser Vaporization of the Prostate

The Nd:YAG laser or diode laser can directly vaporize the periurethral BPH tissue when used in conjunction with special contact tips (available from various manufacturers in numerous designs). Nd:YAG and diode lasers provide excellent hemostasis through dessication and coagulation of the tissue surface, but deep coagulation is not obtained and the ablation rate is low (Daughtry 1992; Daughtry and Rodan 1993; Gilling et al. 1995; Keoghane et al. 1996; Muschter and Perlmutter 1994; Watson 1995). In principle, contact vaporization of the prostate can be obtained with bare fibers (e.g., the Ho:YAG laser) or with side-firing probes designed for noncontact use, but this is less efficient and more time-consuming.

The treatment is performed through a constant-flow urethrocystoscope. The contact tip is positioned in contact with the apical prostatic tissue and advanced to the bladder neck while gentle pressure is applied. Repeating this maneuver in the same position and various other positions can ablate the tissue to a depth of up to 1–2 mm.

The power output is 40–100 W. The tissue can be vaporized to a depth of 2 mm and coagulated to a depth of 1–2 mm.

Transurethral Laser Coagulation of the Prostate (Fig. 4.42)

Various techniques and delivery systems are available for transurethral laser coagulation, also loosely referred to as transurethral laser ablation of the

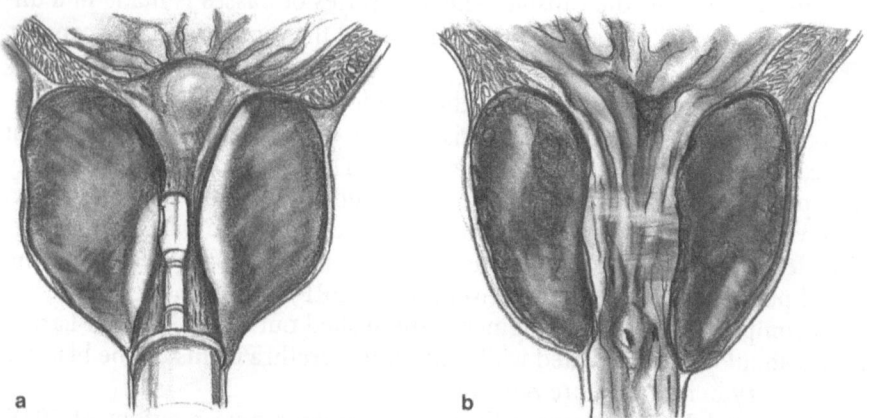

Fig. 4.42. a Side-firing technique. **b** Status following transurethral laser treatment of prostatic adenoma

prostate or laser prostatectomy. All the techniques involve noncontact Nd:YAG laser application to the periurethral prostatic tissue using a deflecting mechanism that usually delivers the laser energy at a 90° angle to the tissue surface. The deflection may be accomplished with bare or balloon-enclosed prisms, metal deflecting dishes, or with fiber tips beveled to a prismatic geometry and protected by glass or metal caps.

Transurethral Ultrasound-Guided Laser-Induced Prostatectomy (TULIP). In the TULIP system the laser fiber is coupled to a right-angle deflecting prism integrated into a urethral probe that contains two ultrasound transducers (Fig. 4.43). The transducers provide the operator with a real-time sector image of the prostatic area that is within the path of the laser beam. Endoscopic visual guidance is not employed. The balloon enclosing the fiber tip serves several functions: it provides a fluid standoff that protects the delivery system, it can lightly compress the adjacent prostatic tissue, and it maintains a constant, predefined distance between the applicator and the tissue surface (Assimos et al. 1991; McCullough 1991; Roth and Aretz 1991; Schulze et al. 1993; Muschter and Hofstetter 1994a).

The delivery system can be mounted on a pistol-grip handle that allows precise control of the axial and radial position of the beam so that laser energy can be applied in a specified pattern to all portions of the prostatic urethra.

After an initial trial pullthrough of the urethral probe, the laser beam is applied to the bladder neck and withdrawn toward the prostatic apex under ultrasound guidance. The pass length is up to 1 cm, depending on the size of the adenoma. After a pause equal to 1.5 times the application time, another pass is made in the next position. An alternating right-left pattern of laser passes is recommended, starting at 3 o'clock and proceeding to the 9, 4, 8, 5, 7, and 6 o'clock positions.

The power output is 35–40 W, the pull rate 0.1–1 mm/s, the depth of penetration 6–15 mm.

Visual/Endoscopic Laser Ablation of the Prostate (VLAP, ELAP, LAP). This technique employs conventional urethrocystoscopes or specially designed laser cystoscopes for the laser ablation of prostatic tissue under visual or endoscopic guidance.

Delivery systems that use a metal reflector for beam deflection may be destroyed if brought into contact with the tissue and should be held stationary when lasing is performed (fixed position lasing).

The beam is applied to the bladder neck at various sites from 2 to 5 o'clock and from 7 to 11 o'clock (lithotomy position) and moved toward the prostatic apex. In each case the beam should be directed toward the main mass of the adenoma. An enlarged median lobe is lased in a more posterior direction at the 5 to 7 o'clock position (Cammack et al. 1993; Costello et al. 1992a,b; Cowles 1992; Cowles et al. 1995; Johnson et al. 1991, 1992; Kabalin 1993; Kabalin et al. 1995, 1996a,b).

An adequate number of laser passes should be used. Many authors recommend a four-point pattern (e.g., at 2, 4, 8, and 10 o'clock) augmented by a second series of passes if the prostate is longer than 2.5 cm. This may leave portions of the adenoma untreated, however, and it is better to space the passes at closer intervals even if this creates a degree of overlap. "Overtreatment" is not hazardous and does not cause adverse side effects; it merely increases the duration of the procedure (Kollmorgen et al. 1996; Muschter and Hofstetter 1994; Perlmutter and Muschter 1994).

Systems in which the beam is deflected with an obliquely beveled fiber tip can usually withstand brief tissue contact without tip destruction, so they can be moved during laser application.

During treatment the laser probe is drawn outwards from the bladder neck toward the prostatic apex ("pulling"). This maneuver is repeated in the next position.

In an alternative technique, called "painting" or "scanning," the probe is rocked slowly back and forth as it is drawn from the bladder neck to the apex, sweeping the beam through a whole sector. A rotating or helical motion can also be used.

In all cases the laser pass should start at the bladder neck and end at the apex (Stein 1992). It is important to move the light guide very slowly to ensure that the desired depth of coagulation is achieved in every area (Perlmutter and Muschter 1994).

The following principles apply regardless of the type of laser probe or application technique that is used:

- It is essential to maintain an adequate safety margin of approximately 1 cm from the bladder sphincter.
- Constant irrigation is maintained during treatment to cool the tissues and improve vision.

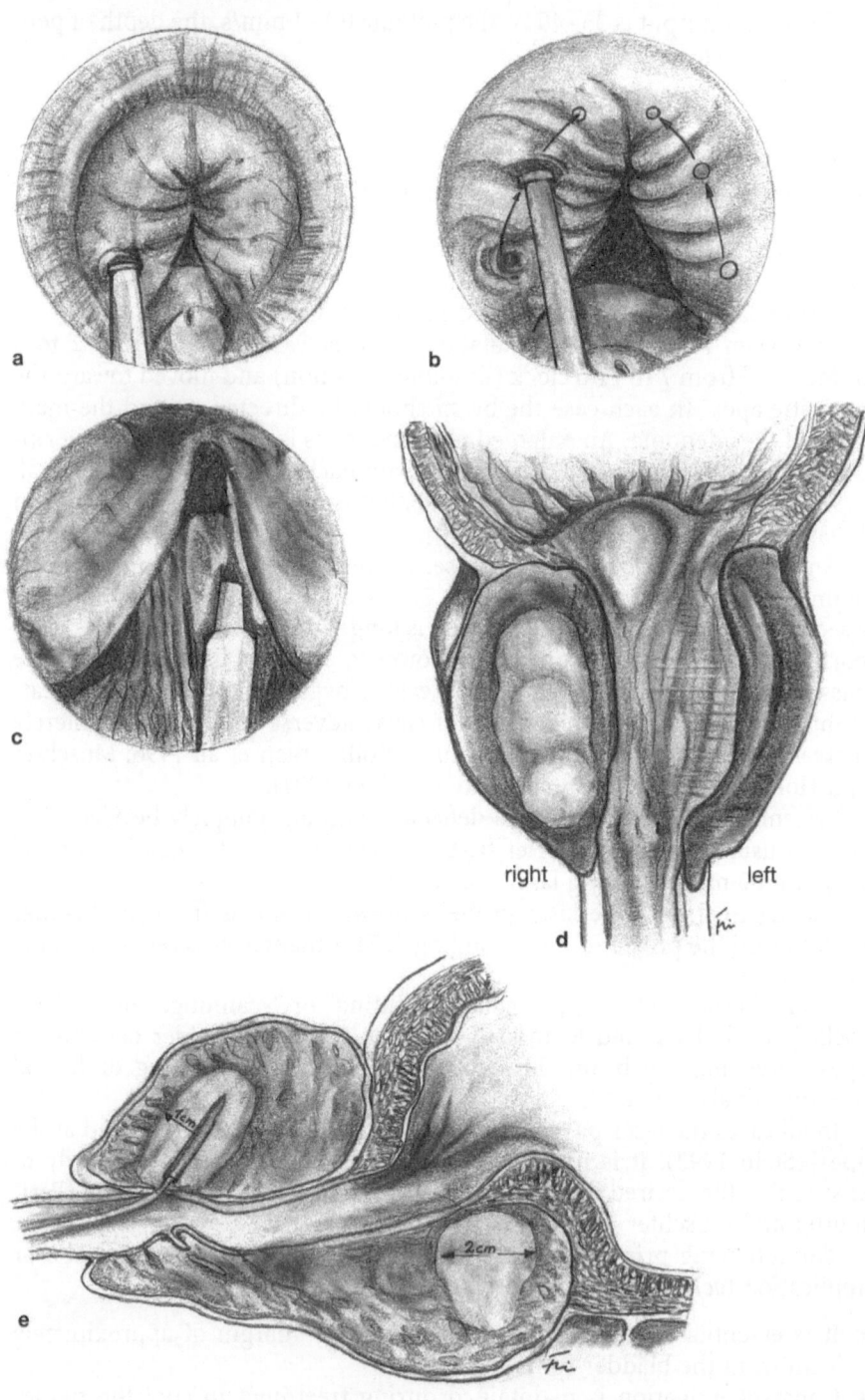

◀ **Fig. 4.43 a–e.** Interstitial laser coagulation of prostatic hyperplasia. **a** The laser probe is placed at the level of the seminal colliculus in the right lateral lobe of the prostate. **b** The probe is moved to a new position in the right lateral lobe. The insertion points lie on an imaginary center line ascending toward the bladder. **c** Treatment of the median lobe. **d** Appearance of the right lobe after three-point interstitial laser therapy. The left lobe illustrates the contraction and resorption of a hyperplastic lobe six weeks after laser treatment. **e** Lateral view shows the position of the laser probe in the hyperplastic prostate (sagittal section)

- The carbonization that occurs with a high power output or prolonged exposure produces surface vaporization but does not increase the penetration depth or enlarge the ablated area.
- Power output: 30–60 W.
- Exposure time: 60–90 s with fixed position lasing, continuous with a moving probe; pull rate: 0.1–1 mm/s.
- Depth of penetration: 6–15 mm.

Transurethral Laser Ablation/Laser Vaporization (TULAP, TUEP). Laser energy that is is delivered at a high power density (high power output from a probe with minimal beam divergence or a very short standoff distance) can vaporize tissue even when a noncontact technique is used. This is time-consuming, however, so noncontact vaporization at a high power density should generally be combined with coagulation, both to achieve the primary relief of bladder outlet obstruction and to induce necrosis and secondary sloughing (Childs 1994; Gilling et al. 1995; Gottfried et al. 1995; Muschter and Perlmutter 1994; Narayan et al. 1995; Perlmutter and Muschter 1994; Shanberg et al. 1994).

Coagulation should always be performed first. Once the surface starts to carbonize, all the laser energy is absorbed at the tissue surface. While this produces vaporization, it prevents any further deep coagulation, much as in contact laser vaporization.

A conventional urethrocystoscope or laser cystoscope is used. Continuous irrigation is necessary to cool the tissues and maintain vision.

The application technique for coagulation is the same as in VLAP. Either an Nd:YAG laser or diode laser can be used, preferably in conjunction with a side-firing probe.

These laser can also be used for subsequent vaporization, or a KTP or Ho:YAG laser can be used (CELAP). The energy can be delivered through a side-firing system or bare fiber, which may be applied in a punctate pattern or may be moved during laser application.

Vaporization requires high power outputs of 60–100 W using a continuous beam.

Interstitial Laser Coagulation of the Prostate

For interstitial laser treatment, the delivery system is inserted directly into the tissue so that the laser energy is applied from inside rather than through the tissue surface. Laser energy that is emitted in a circular pattern can coagulate large tissue volumes, with thermal conduction further increasing the efficacy of the treatment. Volumes of virtually any size can be coagulated by multiple applications.

Unlike transurethral coagulation, ILC usually does not damage the urethra. Generally the necrotic tissue does not communicate with the urethral lumen, so it is not sloughed. The bulk of the adenoma is reduced through atrophic processes and, to a small degree, cicatricial processes (Hofstetter 1991, 1992a,b; Muschter 1994; Muschter and Hofstetter 1992, 1994a,b; 1995a,b; Muschter et al. 1992a,b, 1993, 1996a,b).

Nd:YAG and diode lasers are used with diffusor tips or ITT probes (Frank and Hessel 1990; Hessel and Frank 1990) designed to produce a specific interstitial emission pattern that may be diffuse and homogeneous, diffuse and nonhomogeneous, or may have the shape of a hollow cone (Fig. 4.45). The zone of coagulation necrosis usually coincides in position and extent with the length of the probe. The radius depends on the light guide, the laser parameters, and tissue parameters.

Power output: the initial power output should be high to produce a rapid temperature rise for coagulating the vessels (while keeping just below the carbonization threshold). The output is then reduced in stages by a preset program or adjusted through optical temperature feedback (to maintain the desired temperature).

In the standard Nd:YAG laser program, the power output is stepped down from 20/15/10 W (30 s each) to 7 W (90 s), for a total exposure time of 3 min (Dornier Fibertome with ITT probe). In the standard program for the 830-nm diode laser, the power output is reduced from 10/7.4 W to 5 W over a period of 4 min (Indigo 830 with diffusor tip).

In the high-power program for the Nd:YAG laser, the wattage is decreased from 50 W to 16 W over a period of 1 min (Dornier Fibertome with ITT probe). The high-power program for the 830-nm diode laser starts at 20 or 15 W and uses a feedback system to raise the temperature to a preset value of 85°–100 °C. The power output is automatically adjusted over a total treatment time of 3 min (Indigo 830 with diffusor tip).

Coagulation volume ranges from about 3–5 ml per application in the standard program to about 8 ml per application in the high-power program.

Rectal temperature should always be monitored during ILC (we use the Hofstetter double-balloon catheter with thermosensors; see Fig. 4.44c).

Transurethral Approach. In the transurethral approach (Fig. 4.43a–e), the probe is inserted into the prostatic tissue under visual guidance through a conventional urethrocystoscope, preferably with a special ILC attachment, or through a compact cystoscope with a small working channel to ensure accurate probe positioning. The cap of the ITT probe is completely buried in the prostatic tissue, while the diffusor tip is inserted to the mark. The junction between the optical fiber and cap on the ITT probe or the mark on the diffusor tip defines the boundary of scattering processes in the tissue, ensuring that retrograde coagulation does not occur. After an application is completed, the probe is withdrawn and moved to next position. The number of applications in a given lobe depends on the size of the gland. Undertreatment should be avoided. Too many applications may waste time but are not harmful.

Starting apically just proximal to the external sphincter, the laser probe is inserted at the maximum practical angle of about 25°–35° in thé coronal plane relative to the long axis of the urethra. The insertion points are located at 9–11 o'clock and 1–3 o'clock (lithotomy position).

In the sagittal plane, the probe should be positioned roughly parallel to the urethra in a craniocaudal or slightly anterior orientation (not angled posteriorly). A fan-shaped pattern is useful for large lobes (9–11 o'clock, 7–9 o'clock, 1–3 o'clock, 3–5 o'clock).

The probe is moved about 0.5–1 cm closer to the bladder neck for each additional application. This spacing should produce overlapping zones of coagulation.

The median lobe is treated with single or multiple probe insertions directed toward the bladder lumen. The probe should not be inserted below the level of the trigone.

Percutaneous Transperineal Approach. In the transperineal approach (Fig. 4.44), an aiming device is used to insert the probe into the prostate under transrectal ultrasound guidance. This technique allows for the precise targeting of designated sites. The number of applications depends on the size and configuration of the prostate. The probe is inserted with the aid of a special trocar needle.

Transrectal ultrasound imaging is performed in the coronal and sagittal planes. The target sites are selected to produce an overlapping pattern of laser-induced lesions (the insertions are spaced at intervals of about 1 cm radially and 0.5 cm axially).

After the needle has been inserted and the trocar removed, the laser probe is advanced to the same position in the sheath previously occupied by the trocar. Then the sheath is withdrawn, leaving the probe in place.

Other Techniques

Other experimental techniques described in the literature have not assumed clinical importance (Hardie et al. 1990; Kandel et al. 1986; Watson et al. 1991).

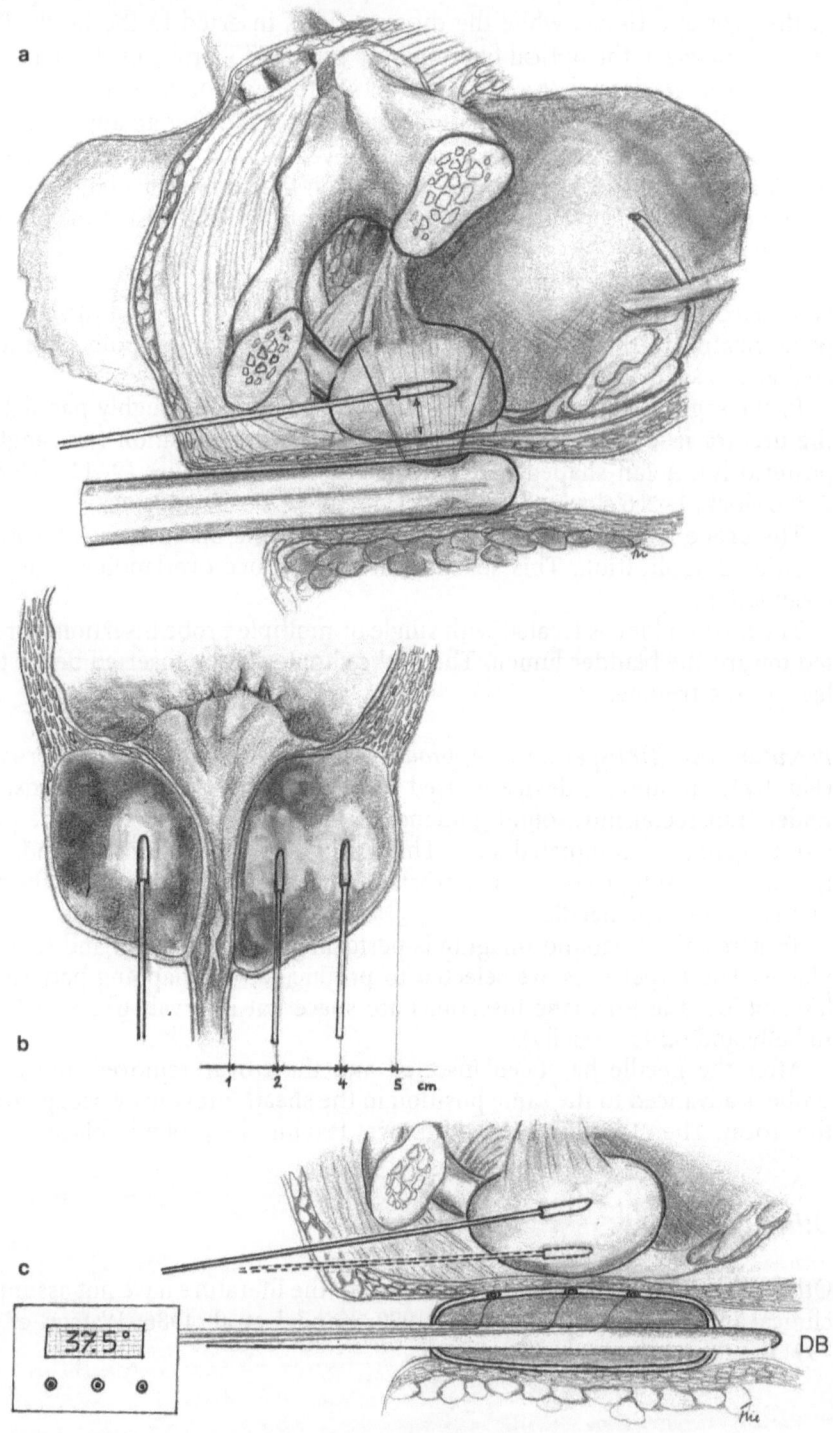

◀ **Fig. 4.44. a** The position of the laser probe in the prostate is monitored by transrectal ultrasound (sagittal section). **b** Necrotic areas within the prostate correspond to the position of the laser probes (cross section). **c** A double-balloon catheter with thermo-sensors (*DB*) is placed within the rectum to monitor the temperature distribution during interstitial laser application

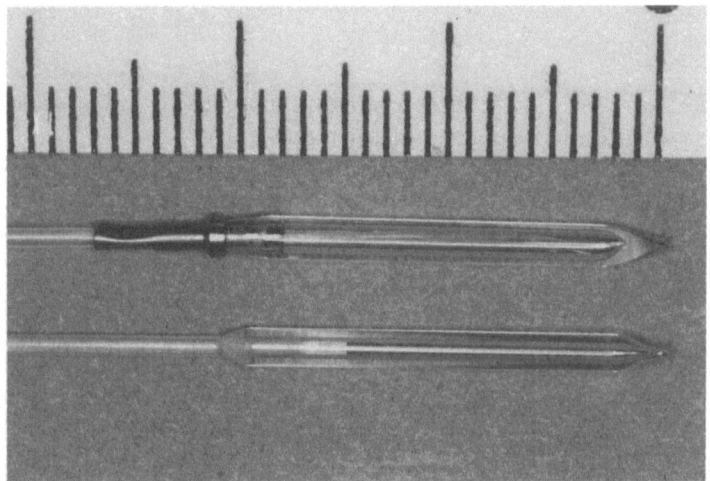

Fig. 4.45. Laser probes for interstitial laser application

Advantages and Disadvantages Compared with Operative Methods

The main advantage of laser prostate surgery over conventional operative methods is a reduction of intra- and perioperative morbidity. Generally these techniques can be used even in high-risk patients. There is significantly less blood loss, and laser surgery eliminates the risk of embolization and associated cardiac risks. Generally the bladder neck can be preserved, so retrograde ejaculation can be avoided. There are differences among the various techniques, however. The more invasive the procedure (e.g., laser resection) and the more aggressive the treatment of the bladder neck, the greater the likelihood of objectionable side effects. Coagulative procedures, especially interstitial coagulation, are associated with very low morbidity.

Most laser surgery can be performed under local anesthesia. Many procedures can be performed on an ambulatory basis, and if hospitalization is required, the stay is generally shorter than with operative methods. Despite the relatively high acquisition costs for delivery systems and other equipment, the overall treatment costs are probably less.

The main disadvantage of coagulative laser surgery is the time delay between treatment and response. Very rarely, it may take 1–2 months to obtain a significant positive response, and occasionally cystoscopy can still detect necrotic residues at 6 months. However, the majority patients do at least as well shortly after surgery as before, and their symptoms continue to improve with passage of time. The protracted response results from the initial hardening of the tissue by coagulation, thermal edema, and the need for eventual sloughing (transurethral ablation) or absorption (ILC) of the necrotic tissues. In the most cases you can avoid disadvantages by bladder neck-incision.

Follow-up

The diagnostic procedures applied preoperatively are also used to monitor or measure the response to laser treatment.

Until the suprapubic bladder catheter (usually placed at operation) is removed, a close watch is kept on urinary output, and prophylaxis or treatment for urinary tract infection is provided as needed. Irritative symptoms that may arise in the early postoperative period are treated symptomatically.

Follow-up examinations are scheduled at 1, 3, and 6 months. The definitive outcome of the treatment cannot be assessed before 3 months.

Contraindications

Laser treatment is contraindicated in patients with an active, untreated genitourinary infection. Some associated disorders (e.g., urethral strictures, bladder stones) can be treated in the same sitting, while others constitute a relative contraindication (e.g., bladder tumors). Certain techniques may not be appropriate in patients with very large prostates, but the cutoff point is determined individually based on the absolute size and configuration of the prostate, the degree of obstruction, and the quality of the bladder.

4.8.2
Prostatic Carcinoma

The techniques described above would be useful as a follow-up to TUR or as an alternative palliative measure to relieve bladder outlet obstruction in patients with prostate cancer (Muschter 1994). The curative laser treatment of localized prostatic carcinoma is still considered experimental.

References

Assimos DG, McCullough DL, Woodruff RD, Harrison LH, Hart LJ, Li WJ (1991) Canine transurethral laser-induced prostatatectomy. J Endourol 5:145–149
Beisland HO (1990) Laserbehandlung des lokalisierten Prostatakarzinoms. In: Staehler G, Fabricius PG (eds). Das Prostatakarzinom. Diagnostik und Therapie. Springer, Berlin Heidelberg New York, pp 97–101

Böwering R, Hofstetter AG, Keiditsch E, Frank F (1979) Irradiation of prostatic carcinoma by neodymium-YAG laser. In: Optics and photonics applied to medicine. SPIE Proc 211, pp 16–20

Cammack JT, Motamedi M, Torres JH, Orihuela E, Cowan D, Warren MM (1993) Endoscopic ND:YAG laser coagulation of the prostate: comparison of lower power versus high power. J Urol 149:215A

Childs SJ (1994) Ablation of prostate tissue at high power density. SPIE Proc 2129:8–14

Camey M, Le Duc A (1980) Preliminary study of the action of the YAG laser on canine prostatic adenoma and experimental urethral stenosis. Eur Urol 6:175–179

Costello AJ, Bowsher WG, Bolton DM, Braslis KG, Burt J (1992a) Laser ablation of the prostate in patients with benign prostatic hypertrophy. Br J Urol 69:603–608

Costello AJ, Johnson DE, Bolton DM (1992b) Nd:YAG laser ablation of the prostate as a treatment for benign prostatic hypertrophy. Lasers Surg Med 12:121–124

Cowles RS (1992) A prospective randomized study comparing transurethral resection of the prostate and visual laser ablation of the prostate. Lasers Surg Med 4 [Suppl]:79

Cowles RS III, Kabalin JN, Childs S, Lepor H, Dixon C, Stein B, Zabbo A (1995) A prospective randomised comparison of transurethral resection to visual laser ablation of the prostate for the treatment of benign prostatic hyperplasia. Urology 46:155–161

Daughtry JD (1992) Transurethral contact laser resection of the prostate. J Urol 147 [Suppl] 201A

Daughtry JD, Rodan BA (1993) Transurethral laser prostatectomy: A comparison of contact tip mode and lateral-firing free beam mode. J Clin Laser Med Surg 11:21–28

Frank F, Hessel S (1990) Technische Voraussetzungen für die interstitielle Thermotherapie mit dem Nd:YAG Laser. Lasermedizin 0:36–40

Gilling PJ, Cass CB, Cresswell MD, Fraundorfer MR (1996) Holmium laser resection of the prostate: preliminary results of a new method for the treatment of benign prostatic hyperplasia. Urology 47:48–51

Gilling PJ, Cass CB, Malcolm AR, Fraundorfer MR (1995) Combination holmium and Nd:YAG laser ablation of the prostate: initial clinical experience. J Endourol 9:151–153

Gottfried HW, Frohneberg D, de la Rosette JJMCH, Lawrence W, Hautmann RE (1995) Transurethral laser ablation of prostate (TULAP). Experience of a European multicenter study using ultraline fiber. J Urol 153:230A

Hardie EM, Stone EA, Spaulding KA, Cullen JM (1990) Subtotal canine prostatatectomy with the neodymium:yttrium-aluminium-garnet laser. Vet Surg 19:348–355

Hessel S, Frank F (1990) Technical prerequisites for interstitial thermotherapy using the Nd:YAG laser. In: Katzir A (ed) Optical fibers in medicine V. SPIE Proc 1201, pp 233–238

Hofstetter AG (1991) Interstitielle Thermokoagulation (ITK) von Prostatatumoren. Lasermedizin 7:179

Hofstetter AG (1992) Laser in der Urologie: neuere Entwicklungen und Forschungsprojekte. Lasermedizin 8:69–72

Hofstetter AG, Muschter R, Hessel S, Keiditsch E (1992) Laser induced thermotherapy in benign prostatic hyperplasia – state of the art. Medtech 3:67

Johnson DE, Costello AJ, Wishnow KI (1991) Transurethral laser prostatectomy using a right-angle laser delivery system. Lasers Surg Med 3 [Suppl]:76

Johnson DE, Price RE, Cromeens DM (1992) Pathological changes occuring in the prostate following transurethral laser prostatectomy. Lasers Surg Med 12:254–263

Kabalin JN (1993) Laser prostatectomy performed with a right angle firing neodymium:YAG laser fiber at 40 watts power setting. J Urol 150:95–99

Kabalin JN, Gill HS, Bite G (1995) Laser prostatectomy performed with a right-angle firing neodymium:YAG laser fiber at 60 watts power setting: J Urol 153:1502–1505

Kabalin JN, Gill HS, Bite G, Doll S (1996) Neodymium-YAG laser coagulation prostatectomy - 3 years of experience with 227 patients. J Urol 155:181–185

Kabalin JN, Terris MK, Mancianti ML, Fajardo LF (1996) Dosimetry studies utilizing the urolase right-angle firing neodymium:YAG laser fiber in the human prostate. Lasers Surg Med 18:72–80

Kandel LB, Harrison LH, McCullough DL, Boyce WH, Woodruff RP, Dyer RB (1986) Transurethral laser prostatectomy: Creation of a technique for using the neodymium: yttrium aluminum garnet (YAG) laser in the canine model. J Urol 135 [Suppl] 110A

Keoghane SR, Cranston DW, Lawrance KC, Doll HA, Fellows GH, Smith C (1996) The Oxford Laser Prostate Trial: a double-blind randomized controlled trial of contact vaporization of the prostate against transurethral resection; preliminary results. Br J Urol 77:382–385

Kollmorgen TA, Malek RS, Barrett DM (1996) Laser prostatectomy: two and half year's experience with aggressive multifocal therapy. Urology 48:217–222

McCullough DL (1991) This month in investigative urology: transurethral laser treatment of benign prostatic hyperplasia. J Urol 146:1126–1127

McNicholas TA, Carter StC, Wickham JEA, O'Donoghue EPN (1988) YAG laser treatment of early carcinoma of the prostate. Br J Urol 61:239–243

Muschter R (1994) Laser induced interstitial thermotherapy of benign prostatic hyperplasia and prostate cancer. SPIE Proc 2327:287–292

Muschter R, Hofstetter AG (1992) "Thermische" Therapie der benignen Prostatahyperplasie. MMW 134:630–634

Muschter R, Hofstetter AG (1994a) Laserbehandlung der benignen Prostatahyperplasie. Urologe A 33:281–287

Muschter R, Hofstetter AG (1994b) Erfahrungen mit der interstitiellen Laserkoagulation in der Therapie der benignen Prostatahyperplasie. Lasermedizin 10:133–139

Muschter R, Perlmutter AP (1994) The optimization of laser prostatectomy. II. other lasing techniques. Urology 44:856–861

Muschter R, Hofstetter AG (1995a) Interstitial laser therapy outcomes in benign prostatic hyperplasia. J Endourol 9:129–135

Muschter R, Hofstetter AG (1995b) Technique and results of interstitial laser coagulation. World J Urol 13:109–114

Muschter R, Hofstetter AG, Hessel S, Keiditsch E, Rothenberger K-H, Schneede P, Frank F (1992a) Hi-Tech of the prostate: Interstitial laser coagulation of benign prostatic hypertrophy. In: Anderson RR (ed) Laser surgery: advanced characterization, therapeutics, and systems III. SPIE Proc 1643, pp 25–34

Muschter R, Hofstetter AG, Hessel S, Keiditsch E, Schneede P (1992b) Interstitial laser prostatectomy - experimental and first clinical results. J Urol 147 [Suppl]:346A

Muschter R, Hessel S, Hofstetter AG, Keiditsch E, Rothenberger K-H, Schneede P, Frank F (1993) Die interstitielle Laserkoagulation der benignen Prostatahyperplasie. Urologe A 32:273–281

Muschter R, Perlmutter AP, Anson K et al (1995a) Diode lasers for interstitial laser coagulation of the prostate. SPIE Proc 2395:77–82

Muschter R, Zellner M, Hessel S, Hofstetter AG (1995b) Die interstitielle laserinduzierte Koagulation (ILK) der Prostata zur Therapie der benignen Hyperplasie (BPH). Urologe A 34:90–97

Narayan P, Tewari A, Fournier G, Toke A (1995) Impact of prostate size on the outcome of transurethral laser evaporation of the prostate for benign prostatic hyperplasia. Urology 45:776–782

Perlmutter AP, Muschter R (1994) The optimization of laser prostatectomy part I: free beam side fire coagulation. Urology 44:847–855

Roth RA, Aretz HT (1991) Transurethral ultrasound-guided laser-induced prostatectomy (TULIP procedure): a canine prostate feasibility study. J Urol 146:1128–1135

Sander S, Beisland HO (1984) Laser in the treatment of localized prostatic carcinoma. J Urol 132:280–281

Schulze H, Martin W, Engelmann U, Senge T (1993) TULIP- transurethrale ultraschallgeführte laserinduzierte Prostatektomie: eine Alternative zur TURP? Urologe A 32:225–231

Shanberg AM, Tansey LA, Baghdassarian R (1985) The use of the neodymium:YAG laser in prostatotomy. J Urol 133 [Suppl]:196 A

Shanberg AM, Lee IS, Tansey LA, Sawyer DE (1994) Extensive neodymium-YAG photoirradiation of the prostate in men with obstructive prostatism. Urology 43:467–471

Stein B (1992) Transurethral resection of benign prostatic hyperplasia with advanced Nd:YAG laser surgical systems. Heraeus, Hanau

Vahlensieck W, Schoeneich G, Vogel J (1990) Adjuvante transurethrale Laserbehandlung des Prostatakarzinoms mit dem 70° Umlenkprisma. Urologe B 30:231–234

Watson G (1995) Contact laser prostatectomy. World J Urol 13:88–93

Watson GM, Perlmutter A, Shah T (1991) A laser balloon for prostatic outflow obstruction. J Endourol 5 [Suppl]: S90

5 Photodynamic Diagnosis and Therapy of Superficial Bladder Cancer

M. Kriegmair, R. Baumgartner, and A.G. Hofstetter

5.1
Theoretical Principles

Photodynamic diagnosis (PDD) and photodynamic therapy (PDT) are based on the interaction between light (usually laser light), photosensitizing compounds that fluoresce when exposed to certain wavelengths of light, and molecular oxygen in the tissue (Dougherty and Marcus 1992). It has been known since about 1960 that porphyrin mixtures such as hematoporphyrin derivative (HpD) administered by i.v. injection accumulate more selectively in neoplastic tissue than in healthy tissues (Ligson and Baldes 1960). The photodynamic therapy of bladder cancer was first performed in 1975 (Kelly and Shell 1976).

The principle of photodynamic diagnosis and therapy is shown in Fig. 5.1. Two to three days after i.v. administration, the photosensitizer (designated S in the figure) accumulates in the bladder tumor. By that time the concentration of the compound is two to five times higher in the tumor than in healthy surrounding tissues. This selective retention is due mainly to the enhanced ability of tumor cells to bind lipoproteins that are laden with the photosensitizing agent. The relative impairment of vascular and lymphatic drainage in the tumor also contributes to the increased uptake.

Diagnostic and therapeutic photodynamic effects are based on light absorption by the photosensitizing porphyrin mixtures. Exposure to violet light with a wavelength of about 400 nm excites a typical red fluorescence in the porphyrin compounds. Since the intensity of the fluorescence correlates with the local concentration of the compounds, the fluorescence provides a conspicuous marker for the visual identification of neoplastic tissue. Ideally, tumors that are not yet detectable endoscopically are rendered visible to the unaided eye.

In addition to their role as diagnostic agents, porphyrins can also be applied therapeutically. In the treatment of bladder tumors, porphyrin photosensitizers are activated by exposing the bladder to red laser light at a wavelength of 630 nm. Although this wavelength is weakly absorbed by porphyrins, it is used because of its high tissue penetration of 3–5 mm, which is 20 to 30 times greater than the penetration depth of violet light. Even so, photodynamic therapy is suitable only for the destruction of superficial tumors.

Fig. 5.1. Principle of photodynamic diagnosis and therapy

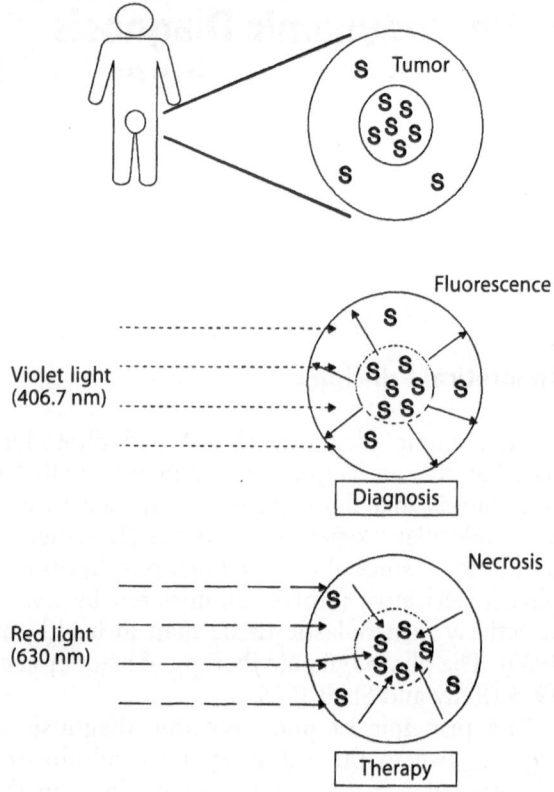

The mechanism of action of PDT is based on the transfer of energy from the excited photosensitizer to oxygen molecules. This leads to the release of a highly reactive oxygen species (singlet oxygen) that destroys vital cellular structures such as mitochondrial membranes. Studies have also shown an extensive disruption of the tumor capillary system by PDT. The photodynamically induced injuries to cells and vascular channels ultimately lead to the death of the cell. PDT also induces a prolonged, presumably nonspecific stimulation of the immune system that probably enhances the therapeutic effect (Nseyo et al. 1990). All these mechanisms make PDT an excellent modality for the curative treatment of superficial malignancies.

Therapeutic photosensitizers selectively accumulate in tumor tissue and, when excited by light absorption, not only exert cytotoxic effects but also show fluorescent emission. This forms the basis of "fluorescent cystoscopy," which permits the visual detection of otherwise endoscopically occult precancerous lesions, micropapillary tumors, and carcinoma in situ.

When systemically administered photosensitizers such as Photofrin or Photosan-3 are used for the fluorescent detection of tumor sites, sophisticated image processing technology is needed to suppress tissue autofluorescence (Baumgartner et al. 1992). This can be avoided by using 5-aminolevulinic acid (ALA), a precursor in the heme biosynthesis pathway. Several enzymatic reactions that occur in mitochondria and cytosol lead to the synthesis of highly pure porphyrin monomers, chiefly protoporphyrin IX. When ALA is instilled into the bladder, it effectively stimulates protoporphyrin synthesis at sites of urothelial neoplasia. This induces an endogenous fluorescence greater than that produced by systemic photosensitizers and of an intensity that is plainly visible on cystoscopic examination (Kriegmair et al. 1992).

5.2
Photodynamic Diagnosis

Indications

The rates of tumor recurrence and progression following the transurethral resection of bladder tumors depend largely on the presence of carcinoma in situ and precancerous lesions (grade I–III dysplasia, atypical hyperplasias, leukoplakia) in the residual mucosa. These flat urothelial lesions are very difficult to detect by conventional endoscopy, and some can occur in quite normal-appearing mucosa (Althausen et al. 1976; Flamm and Dona 1989; Smith et al. 1978). These lesions can be visualized by fluorescent cystoscopy. At present, only the following high-risk subsets of patients are candidates for photodynamic examination of the bladder due to the limited resources available for PDD:

- Patients with more than two recurrences within the past six months
- Patients with a history of carcinoma in situ
- Patients with multifocal tumors
- Patients with positive urine cytology but no endoscopic or histological evidence of tumor

Technique

Photodynamic diagnosis and fluorescent cystoscopy are used for the detection of flat precancerous and malignant lesions that are difficult or impossible to detect by conventional cystoscopy.

For video documentation of the intraoperative findings, the fluorescent images can be recorded with an image intensifier camera that is sensitive to red wavelengths (l>600 nm). Endoscopic findings can be documented with an ordinary color video camera (Fig. 5.2). The procedure starts with the intravesical instillation of 3 % 5-aminolevulinic acid solution buffered to a neutral pH in $NaHCO_3$. The solution should remain in the bladder for at least 1 h, then fluorescent cystoscopy is performed while the interior of the bladder is illuminated with violet laser light. Ordinary UV light can be used as an alternative to the UV laser. Precancerous mucosal lesions and tumors fluoresce a bright red under the UV illumination. These fluorescent sites can be selectively biopsied and subsequently treated by Nd:YAG laser photocoagulation (Fig. 5.3).

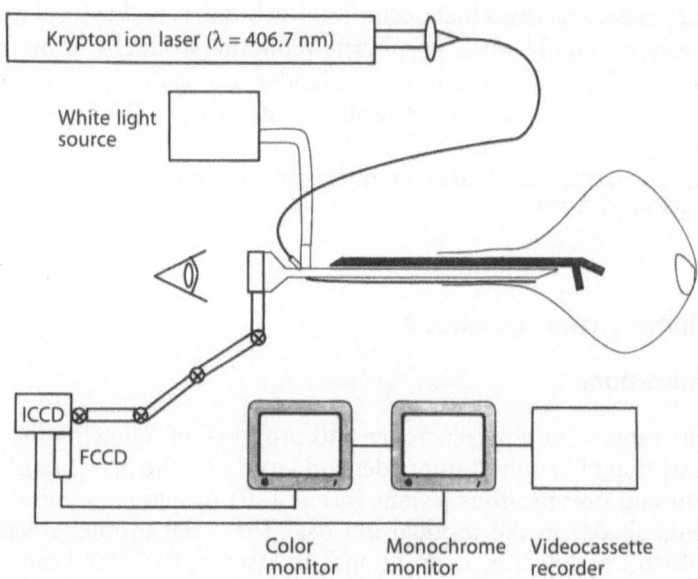

Fig. 5.2. Schematic arrangement of a system for fluorescent cystoscopy with video documentation

Fig. 5.3. Fluorescent cystoscopic view of red fluorescence localized to micropapillary bladder tumors

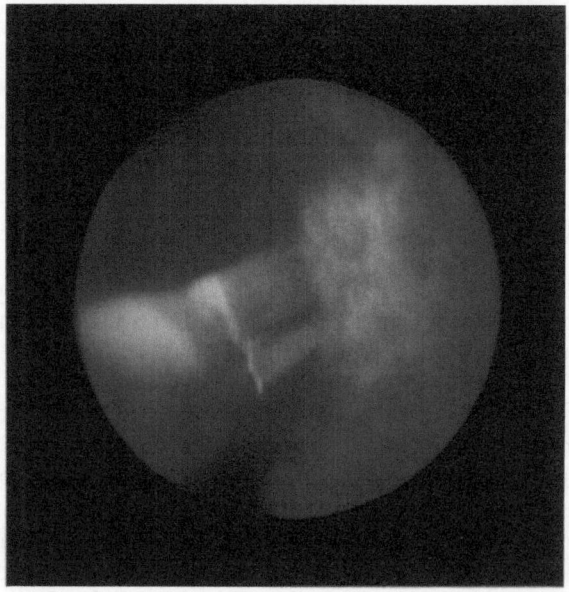

Advantages

- In situ diagnosis of dysplasia, carcinoma in situ, and micropapillary tumors
- Limitation of biopsies to the fluorescent sites
- High sensitivity compared with random biopsy, cytology, and flow cytometry
- Good visibility in blood-tinged irrigant, as violet light is poorly reflected by hemoglobin
- Ability to combine diagnostic fluorescence with Nd:YAG laser coagulation

Disadvantages

- Extra costs due to modified surgical instruments and the instillation of ALA

Contraindications

- Vesicorenal reflux
- Renal function impairment with creatinine >2.5 mg%
- Liver function impairment with bilirubin >3 mg%
- Transaminase levels more than twice the limit of upper normal
- Quick PT <60%, cholinesterase <2000 U/l, GT >60 U/l
- WBC <3500, platelet count <100000
- Pregnancy
- Porphyria or porphyrin allergy

Equipment

Photodynamic diagnosis and therapy are in the clinical testing stage, so equipment is subject to ongoing developments and modifications in the light of clinical experience. The following list reflects the current state of the art:

- Photosensitizing agent:
  - 5-Aminolevulinic acid hydrochloride (Merck)
  - Three percent solution dissolved in $NaHCO_3$ (pH=7)
  - Intravesical instillation of 50 ml
  - Minimum instillation time: 1 h
- Light source:
  - Krypton ion laser or ordinary UV light
  - Wavelengths: $\lambda = 406.7$ nm and 413.5 nm (multiline violet)
  - Power output >300 mW

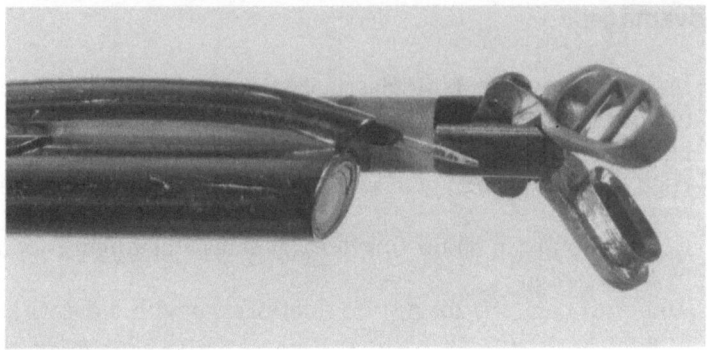

Fig. 5.4. Biopsy forceps used with a Ch 26 constant-flow resectoscope equipped with an integrated fiber for PDD

- Excitation fiber:
  - 500 μm plastic fiber with biconical tip (custom made)
  - Emission angle >60°
  - Power output at fiber tip approx. 200 mW
- Endoscope (Fig. 5.4):
  - Integrated biopsy forceps
  - Integrated excitation fiber (custom made)
- Observation:
  - With the naked eye through the endoscope
- Documentation:
  - Articulated coupling between the endoscope and camera system
  - Color CCD camera for white-light observation
  - CCD intensifier camera for recording fluorescent images
  - Electromechanical relay between the cameras (custom made)
  - Videotape recording system (U-Matic)

5.3
Photodynamic Therapy

Indications

Recurrent superficial bladder cancer is associated with a general carcinogenic predisposition involving all of the urothelial mucosa. Thus, curative treatment in such cases requires integral treatment of the entire mucosa. Traditionally, the only option remaining after unsuccessful chemoprophylaxis, immunoprophylaxis, and BCG instillation therapy has been cystectomy. Photodynamic therapy now offers such patients a final recourse that may allow preservation of the bladder (Kriegmair et al. 1992). The specific indications are as follows:

- Recurrent multifocal carcinoma in situ
- Recurrent multifocal micropapillary tumors (Ta grades I–III)
- Failure of BCG instillation and chemotherapy
- Candidates for radical cystectomy

Technique

Photodynamic therapy starts with the intravenous administration of synthetic porphyrins. Photofrin (2.5 mg/ml) and Photosan-3 (3.3 mg/ml) are in clinical use. These oligomeric mixtures of compounds are composed of porphyrin rings linked by ester bridges. Whole-bladder photoirradiation is performed 48–72 h after i. v. injection of the photosensitizing porphyrin. A continuous-flow cystoscope is passed into the bladder. The constant irrigation ensures unobscured vision and light delivery in these patients, many of whom have had multiple previous operations and a bladder mucosa that is highly susceptible to injury. Light absorption by hemoglobin is reduced, and more homogeneous photoirradiation is obtained.

The inflow pressure of the irrigant (0.9 % NaCl), or the height at which the irrigation reservoir is suspended above the patient, should be just enough to unfold and smoothly distend the bladder wall. The irrigant volume needed to produce this distention is then determined and, along with the power output measured from the spherical tip of the laser fiber, is used to calculate the necessary exposure time (see dosimetry equipment and Table 5.1).

The bladder is refilled using the irrigant pressure previously required for bladder distension, and the spherical fiber tip is positioned at the center of the bladder lumen. Fiber placement is gauged with the aid of a Ch 3 ureteral catheter passed through the fiber channel. The constant-flow cystoscope is then securely mounted on a stand, and the laser is activated for the calculated exposure time.

The following parameters are recommended for the photodynamic therapy of bladder cancer:

- Photosensitizer dose (Photofrin or Photosan-J): 1.5–2 mg/kg b.w
- Energy dose: 15–20 J/cm^2
- Power output at the spherical fiber tip: 1.5–2.5 W
- Bladder distention: 150–220 ml
- Exposure time: 20–60 min

Advantages

- Selective destruction of premalignant and malignant mucosal lesions.
- Opportunity for bladder preservation in patients who have reached the limits of conservative therapy.

Table 5.1. Exposure times for photodynamic therapy of the bladder as a function of light output (L), bladder volume (V), bladder surface area (F), and bladder diameter (d)

V [cm³]	100	120	140	160	180	200	220	240	260	280	300	320	340	360	380
F [cm²]	104	118	130	143	154	165	176	187	197	207	217	226	236	245	254
d [cm²]	5.8	6.1	6.4	6.7	7.0	7.3	7.5	7.7	7.9	8.1	8.3	8.5	8.7	8.8	9.0
L [W]															
1.00	26:03	29:25	32:36	35:38	38:33	41:21	44:04	46:41	49:15	51:45	54:11	56:34	58:54	61:11	63:26
1.20	21:42	24:31	27:10	29:42	32:07	34:27	36:43	38:55	41:03	43:07	45:09	47:08	49:05	50:59	52:51
1.40	18:36	21:01	23:17	25:27	27:32	29:32	31:28	33:21	35:11	36:58	38:42	40:24	42:04	43:42	45:18
1.60	16:17	18:23	20:22	22:16	24:05	25:51	27:32	29:11	30:47	32:20	33:52	35:21	36:49	38:14	39:39
1.80	14:28	16:20	18:07	19:48	21:25	22:58	24:29	25:56	27:22	28:45	30:06	31:25	32:43	33:59	35:14
2.00	13:01	14:42	16:18	17:49	19:16	20:40	22:02	23:21	24:38	25:52	27:05	28:17	29:27	30:35	31:43
2.20	11:50	13:22	14:49	16:12	17:31	18:48	20:02	21:13	22:23	23:31	24:38	25:43	26:46	27:49	28:50
2.40	10:51	12:15	13:35	14:51	16:04	17:14	18:21	19:27	20:31	21:34	22:34	23:34	24:32	25:30	26:26
2.60	10:01	11:19	12:32	13:42	14:49	15:54	16:57	17:57	18:57	19:54	20:50	21:45	22:39	23:32	24:24
2.80	09:18	10:30	11:39	12:44	13:46	14:46	15:44	16:41	17:35	18:29	19:21	20:12	21:02	21:51	22:39
3.00	08:41	09:48	10:52	11:53	12:51	13:47	14:41	15:34	16:25	17:15	18:04	18:51	19:38	20:24	21:09
3.20	08:08	09:12	10:11	11:08	12:03	12:55	13:46	14:35	15:23	16:10	16:56	17:41	18:24	19:07	19:49
3.40	07:40	08:39	09:35	10:29	11:20	12:10	12:58	13:44	14:29	15:13	15:56	16:38	17:19	18:00	18:39
3.60	07:14	08:10	09:03	09:54	10:42	11:29	12:14	12:58	13:41	14:22	15:03	15:43	16:22	17:00	17:37
3.80	06:51	07:44	08:35	09:23	10:09	10:53	11:36	12:17	12:58	13:37	14:15	14:53	15:30	16:06	16:41

Disadvantages

- General photosensitization of the skin for 6–8 weeks. Patients should avoid exposure to direct sunlight for 30 days (Dougherty et al. 1990).
- Development of a contracted bladder (risk <10%) or hydronephrosis (risk <1%).
- Some patient experience significant dysuric complaints, including gross hematuria and suprapubic pain, for 2–4 weeks after treatment.
- There is a theoretical risk of systemic progression due to delay of radical surgery, but so far we have not encountered this problem in a series of 20 patients.

Follow-up

- Cystoscopy, preferably including diagnostic fluorescence and selective biopsy, is performed every three months after PDT.
- Lavage cytology and renal ultrasound are also recommended.

Contraindications

- Invasive bladder cancer (stage T2 or higher)
- Bladder capacity <200 cm^2
- Positive biopsy of the prostatic urethra or prostate
- Impaired renal and/or hepatic function (creatinine >2.5 mg/dl, SGOT, SGPT, alkaline phosphatase more than twice normal limit, total bilirubin >2 mg/dl)
- WBC <3500, platelet count <100 000
- Pregnancy
- Porphyria or allergy to porphyrins

Equipment

Photodynamic diagnosis and therapy are in the clinical testing stage, so equipment is subject to ongoing developments and modifications as more clinical experience is gained. The following list reflects the current state of the art (1993–1994):

- Photosensitizing agent:
  - Photofrin, 2.5 mg/ml
  - Photosan-3, 3.3 mg/ml
  - Dose: 2 mg/kg b.w. by i.v. injection
- Light source:
  - Argon ion laser, pumped dye laser

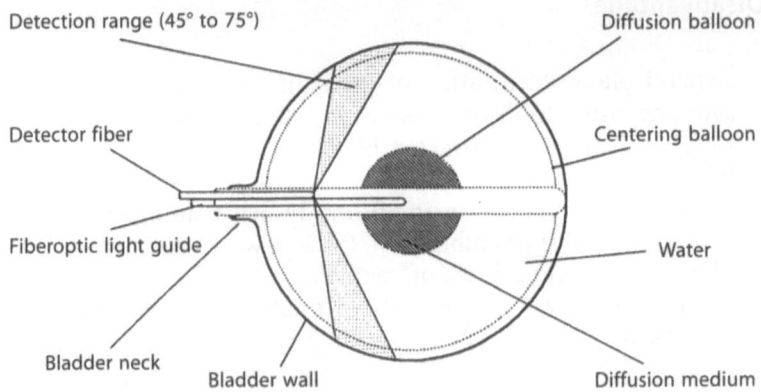

Fig. 5.5. Schematic diagram of a PDT catheter with integrated treatment fiber and dosimetric fiber

- Emission wavelength $\lambda = 630$ nm (should be checked with hand monochromator)
- Continuous power output: 2.7 W (laser system: coherent lambda plus)
- Laser probe:
  - 400 µm quartz fiber coupled to bulb-type emitter (2.5 mm in diameter).
  - Probe is centrally positioned in the bladder with the aid of a ureteral catheter.
  - The endoscope is mounted on a fixed stand.
  - PDT catheter with capacity for on-line dosimetry (Fig. 5.5).
- PDT dosimetry:
  - Bladder surface area calculated from the bladder volume (with smooth distention of the bladder wall).
  - Exposure time calculated from the bladder surface area and light output at the probe tip for a total dose of 151 J/cm^2 (Table 5.1). This is performed with a special wattmeter (custom made) that can be used with diffusely emitting probes. The meter is calibrated by immersing the probe tip in sterile saline solution.
  - Optional: fiber-supported dosimetry unit for individual determination and control of the intracavitary light dose (Marynissen et al. 1989; Pangratz et al., in preparation).

References

Althausen AF, Prout GR Jr, Daly JJ (1976) Noninvasive papillary carcinoma of the bladder associated with carcinoma in situ. J Urol 116:575

Baumgartner R, Kriegmair M, Jocham D, Hofstetter AG, Huber R, Karg O, Haussinger K (1992) Photodynamic diagnosis (PDD) of early stage malignancies – preliminary results in urology and pneumology. In: Mang TT (ed) Physiological monitoring and early detection diagnostic methods. SPE Prog 1641, p 107

Dougherty TJ, Marcus SL (1992) Photodynamic therapy. Eur J Cancer 28A/10:1734

Dougherty TJ, Cooper MT, Mang TS (1990) Cutaneous phototoxic occurrences in patients receiving Photofrin. Lasers Surg Med 10:185

Flamm J, Dona S (1989) The significance of bladder quadrant biopsies in patients with primary superficial bladder cancer. Eur Urol 16:81

Kelly IF, Snell ME (1976) Hematoporphyrin derivative: a possible aid in the diagnosis and therapy of carcinoma of the bladder. J Urol 115:150

Kriegmair M, Baumgartner R, Hofstetter AG (1992) Intravesikale Instillation von Delta-Aminolävulinsaure (ALA) – eine neue Methode zur photodynamischen Diagnostik und Therapie. Lasermedizin 8:83

Kriegmair M, Baumgartner R, Hofstetter AG (1992) Photodynamische Behandlung des oberflächlichen Harnblasenkarzinoms. MMW 134:635

Lipson RL, Baldes EJ (1960) The photodynamic properties of a particular hematoporphyrin derivative. Arch Dermatol 82:508

Marynissen JPA, Jansen H, Star WM (1989) Treatment system for whole-bladder-wall photodynamic therapy with in vivo monitoring and control of light dose rate and dose. J Urol 142:1351

Nseyo UO, Whalen RK, Duncan MR et al (1990) Urinary cytokines following photodynamic therapy for bladder cancer: A preliminary report. Urology 36:167

Pongratz T, Beyer W, Hofstetter AG (in preparation) Lichtdosimetrie für die photodynamische Lasertherapie in der Harnblase. In: Waidelich W (ed) Laser in der Medizin

Smith G, Elton RA, Beynin LL, Newsam JE, Chishol, GD, Hargreave TB (1978) Prognostic significance of biopsy results of normal-looking mucosa in cases of superficial bladder cancer. J Urol 120:57

6 Laser Lithotripsy of Ureteral Stones

A.G. Hofstetter, N. Schmeller, and A. Ehsan

There is a diversity of opinion among international experts on the role of extracorporeal shock wave lithotripsy (ESWL) in the treatment of ureteral stones. While most German authors consider ESWL the method of first choice, we agree with a number of American authors that ureteroscopic lithotripsy is the primary modality, especially for prevesical stones, owing to its rapid efficacy and low invasiveness. We particularly favor the transurethral approach now that a special catheter has been devised enabling most lower and midureteral stones to be destroyed blindly, without the need for ureteroscopic visualization. This technique requires the use of a specially designed pulsed dye laser (Lithognost) with an optical feedback system for automatic stone detection (Bhatta et al. 1990; Dretler 1990; Engelhardt et al. 1988; Hofmann et al. 1990; Hofstetter et al. 1986; Pertusa et al. 1991; Schmeller et al. 1989, 1990, 1991; Weissmüller et al. 1991). Besides the laser, electrohydraulic probes and compressed air-driven impactors can also be used for ureteroscopic lithotripsy (Bagley 1990; Morgenthaler et al. 1990; Schmeller 1991; Segura 1990).

Indications

- Impacted ureteral stones
- Stones that have failed ESWL
- Stones in the lower or middle third of the ureter

Preoperative Studies

- Abdomen plain film, ultrasound, intravenous urogram

Operative Technique

- A ureteral stone with hydronephrosis and fever is initially managed by percutaneous nephrostomy and antibiotics, followed by laser lithotripsy.
- ESWL is indicated for an impacted upper ureteral stone that is not expected to pass spontaneously and is not associated with urinary obstruction or unremitting colic.

- Laser lithotripsy is indicated for stones that fail ESWL or for a lower or midureteral stone that is associated with colicky pain and is not expected to pass spontaneously.
  - *Ureterorenoscopy* (rigid or flexible endoscope, Ch 6.8–8.5) using laser fibers 200–220 µm in diameter and a pulsed dye laser (Lithognost) with automatic stone detection for lithotripsy. This laser can deliver outputs as high as 150 mJ, which is sufficient to destroy more than 90 % of urinary calculi. Besides the pulsed dye laser, the alexandrite and Nd:YAG lasers can also be used. The main disadvantage of the alexandrite laser is that significant erosion of the optical fiber occurs at just 60 mJ. Also, the Nd:YAG laser must be used with an optomechanical coupler in order to generate shock waves. Available optomechanical couplers are too large to use conveniently within the ureter (Pensel et al. 1981). When the ureteroscope is inserted, irrigant should be instilled at a very low flow rate to avoid driving the stone farther up the ureter. Then the closed Dormia basket is advanced past the stone and opened proximal to it. The plastic sheath is removed from the basket to make room for the laser fiber. If the stone breaks up during laser lithotripsy, the larger fragments are captured in the Dormia basket (Fig. 6.1a). The main body of the stone may be carefully extracted, or it may be fragmented into sandlike particles that are allowed to pass spontaneously (Fig. 6.1b).
  - The laser catheter designed by Hofstetter (manufactured by Angiomed) can be inserted cystoscopically into the ureter until it touches the stone (confirmed by contrast or noncontrast radiography; Figs. 6.2, 6.3). The catheter is then withdrawn 2–3 mm, and the laser fiber is advanced and fired. If the laser breaks the stone up into larger fragments, the Dormia basket is advanced to entrap the stone, and laser fragmentation is continued until only sand remains. The basket is withdrawn into the catheter sheath, and the catheter is passed up into the renal pelvis. All instrumentation is then removed from the laser catheter, leaving the sheath within the ureter as a drainage stent. This drainage is necessary only in patients with an impacted stone or patients who have undergone previous ESWL. The catheter sheath can be removed two days later.

Advantages

- Over ESWL: there is immediate stone elimination with unimpeded urinary outflow and no steinstrasse.
- Over open surgery: minimal invasiveness.
- Over the lithoclast and electrohydraulic probes: can be used blindly and does not perforate the ureter.

Fig. 6.1. Ureteroscopic lithotripsy. *Left:* The ureteral stone is
entrapped in the Dormia basket.
Right: The stone is destroyed by
laser-induced shock waves

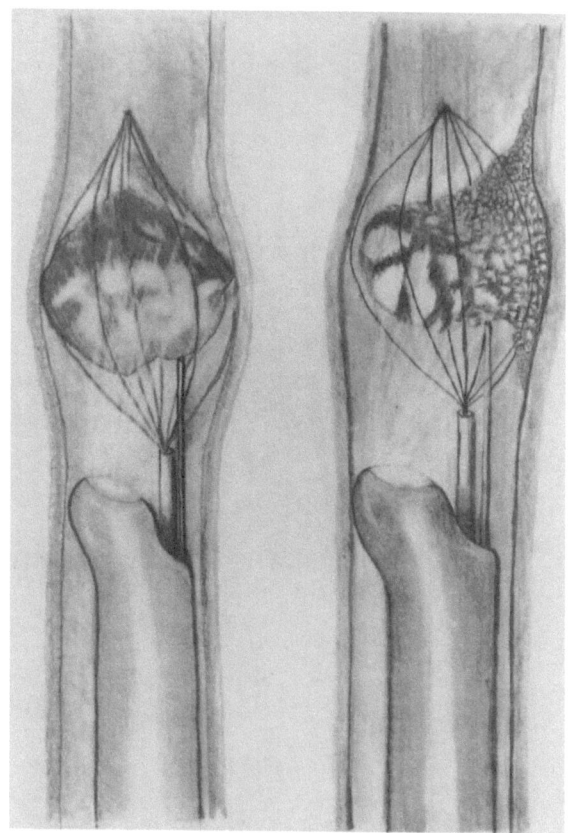

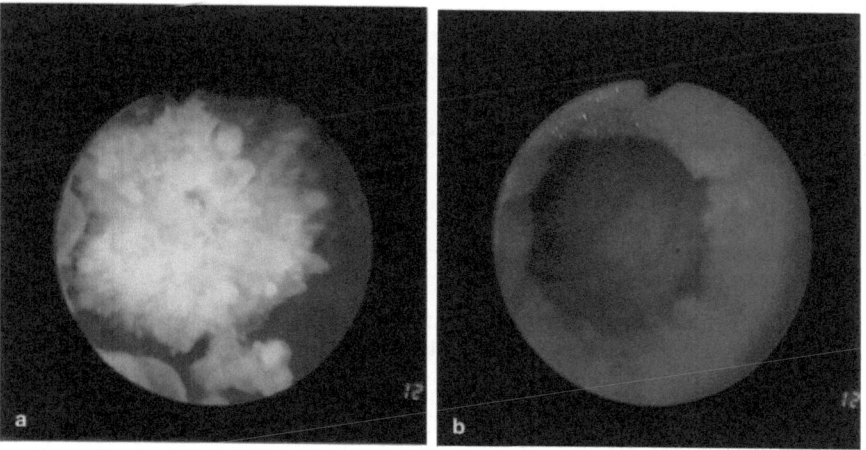

Fig. 6.2. a, b. Impacted ureteral stone: **a** before treatment, **b** after laser lithotripsy

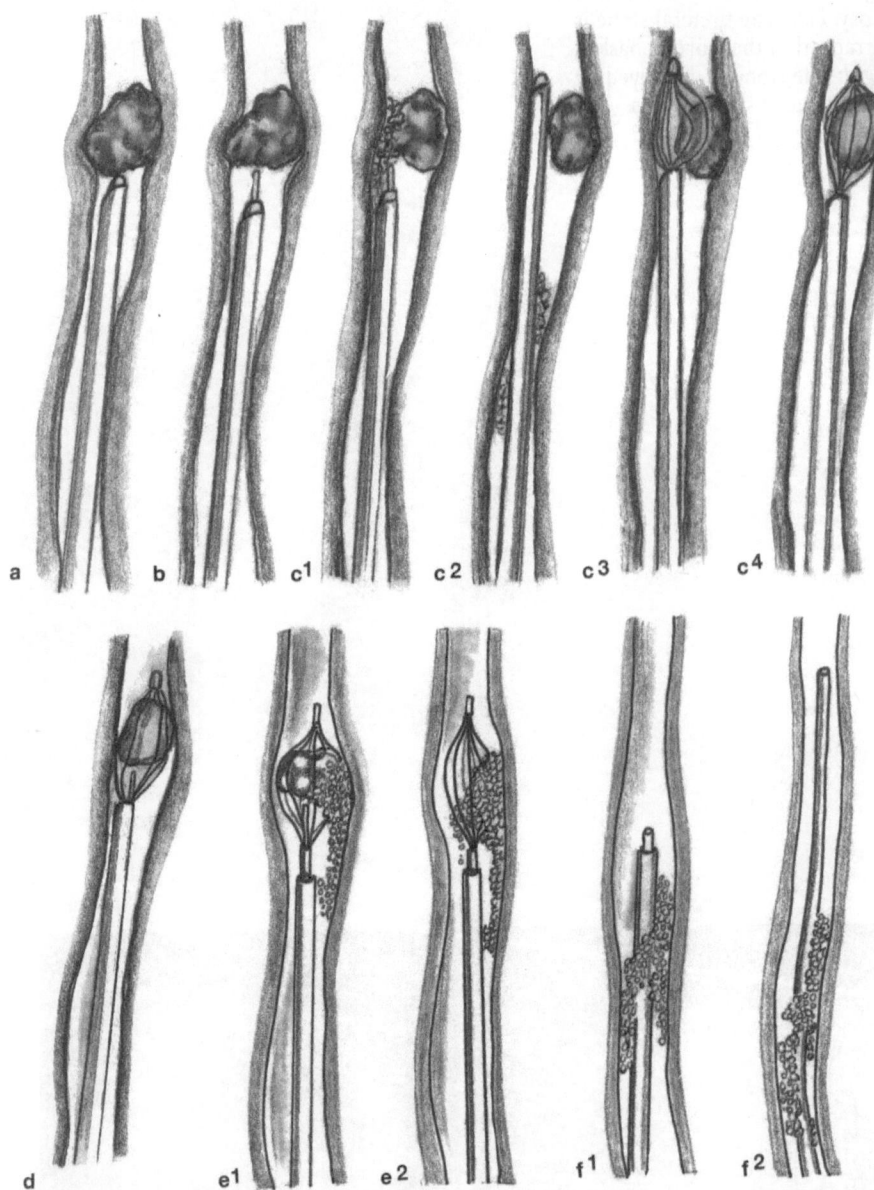

Fig. 6.3a–f. Ureteral stone fragmentation using the laser catheter designed by Hofstetter. **a** The laser catheter is advanced until it touches the stone. **b** The catheter is withdrawn 2–3 mm, and the laser fiber is advanced. **c** The stone is destroyed by the laser-induced shock wave; larger fragments are captured in the Dormia basket. **d** The laser fiber is advanced, and additional shock waves are applied. **e** The immobilized stone is fragmented into small particles by the laser-induced shock waves. **f** After the stone has been destroyed, all instrumentation is removed from the laser catheter, and the sheath is advanced cephalad to drain the renal pelvis

Contraindications

- Intrarenal stones should be managed by ESWL or percutaneous lithola-
paxy, depending on the size of the stone. For staghorn calculi, both procedures should be combined.

Instrumentation

The flashlamp-pumped dye laser with automatic stone detection (Lithognost) has yielded very good clinical results. Alexandrite lasers are also
available, but excessive fiber erosion can limit the performance of these systems. Nd:YAG laser systems must be used with optomechanical couplers for
maximum efficiency, but the size of these devices makes them difficult to
use in the ureter.

The dye laser that we developed in collaboration with the Telemit com-
pany (Lithognost) uses as its lasing medium Rhodamine XG, which emits at
a wavelength of 594 nm. Our laser employs an automatic feedback system
that can discriminate stone from soft tissue. Laser light reflected from the
surface of the target during the first 10 ns of the laser pulse is transmitted
back through the laser-emitting quartz fiber and is analyzed. Basic studies
(Engelhardt et al. 1988; Schmeller et al. 1990) have shown that biological tissue can be accurately differentiated from stone by analysis of the remission
spectrum. If a "stone signal" is not received from the targeted matter, the
laser pulse is interrupted at once by a polarizing filter (90° rotation of the
polarization plane). By that time only about 10 % of the total energy of the
laser pulse has been emitted, so there is no injury to the ureteral wall.

The *alexandrite laser* operates at a wavelength of 755 nm and has a maximum energy output of 60–70 mJ. Because this wavelength is strongly
absorbed by a dark surface, the alexandrite laser is best suited for the fragmentation of pure oxalate monohydrate stones (Schmeller 1991). Pale calculi absorb little energy at this wavelength and are not efficiently fragmented.

The pulsed *Nd:YAG laser* must be used with an optomechanical coupler
to generate shock waves for lithotripsy. Attempts to polish a spherical lens
on the end of the quartz fiber have been unsuccessful due to poor mechanical stress tolerance (Hofmann et al. 1990; Schmeller et al. 1989, 1991;
Weissmüller et al. 1991).

References

Bagley DH (1990) Removal of upper urinary tract calculi with flexible ureteropyeloscopy. Urology 35:412–416

Bhatta KM, Rosen DJ, Flotte TJ, Dretler SP, Nishioka NS (1990) Effects of shielded and
unshielded laser and electrohydraulic lithotripsy on rabbit bladder. J Urol
143:857–860

Dretler SP (1990) An evaluation of ureteral laser lithotripsy: 225 consecutive patients. J Urol 143:267-272

Engelhardt R, Meyer W, Hering P (1988) Spectroscopy during laser-induced shock wave lithotripsy. Spie Proc 906, p 63

Hofmann R, Hartung R, Schmidt-Kloiber H, Reichel E (1990) Laserlithotripsie mit dem Neodym-YAG Laser. Urologe A 29:300-303

Hofstetter AG, Frank F, Kreiditsch E, Wondruzek T (1985) Intrakorporale, laserinduzierte Stoßwellen-Lithotripsie. Laser 1:155-156

Morgentaler A, Bridge SS, Dretler SP (1990) Management of the impacted ureteral calculus. J Urol 143:263-266

Pensel J, Frank F, Rothenberger KH, Hofstetter AG, Unsold E (1981) Destruction of urinary calculi by Nd:YAG laser irradiation. In: Kaplan (ed) Laser surgery, vol 10. Academic, pp 4-6

Pertusa C, Albisu A, Acha M, Blasco M, Llarena R, Arregui P (1991) Lithotropsy with the alexandrite laser: our initial 100 clinical cases. Eur Urol 20:269-271

Schmeller N (1991) Stone fragmentation capacities of different lasers and EHL in monohydrate, cystine and struvite urinary calculi. In: Jocham D, Thüroff JW, Rübben H (eds) Investigative urology 4, Springer, Berlin Heidelberg New York, pp 212-215

Schmeller N, Hofstetter AG, Kriegmair M, Frank F, Wondrazek F (1989) Intrakorporale Stoßwellenlithotropsie mit den Nd:YAG Laser. Fortschr Med 108:559-562

Schmeller N, Kriegmair M, Liedl B, Hofstetter AG, Muschter R, Thomas S, Knipper A (1990) Laserlithotripsie mit automatischer Abschaltung bei Gewebekontakt. Urologie A 29:309-312

Schmeller N, Liedl B, Kriegmair M, Hofstetter AG (1991) Elektrohydraulische im Vergleich zur laserinduzierten Lithotripsie von Harnleitersteinen. Urologe A 30:A64

Segura JW (1990) Surgical management of urinary calculi. Semin Nephrol 10:53-63

Weissmüller J, Schafhauser W, Schrott KM, Hochberger JH, Ell C (1991) Laserlithotripsie von Harnleitersteinen. Eigene Erfahrungen. Urologe A 30:333-336

7 Future Prospects

A.G. HOFSTETTER

The use of lasers in medicine is opening up a broad new area of surgical capabilities that include procedures on the normal and neoplastic cell itself. Besides the effects of various laser wavelengths on the physiological processes in cells, one can easily imagine performing selective manipulations on intracellular organelles, cell nuclei, and even DNA. Such applications could go well beyond "optical forceps" to photodynamic interventions such as using viral vectors to introduce photosensitizing agents or photosensitizing cytostatic drugs into the DNA, sensitizing it to specific wavelengths of laser light. Moreover, we have scarcely begun to explore the diagnostic capabilities of gas analysis by Raman spectroscopy, x-ray lasers for the ultrastructural analysis of cells, and techniques for the photoablation and photodisruption of molecular structures.

Besides potential laser applications in molecular biology and genetic engineering (laser microbeam), there is still room for the improvement and expansion of current laser surgical techniques. These advances depend partly on the future development of fiberoptic technology, which first enabled the endoscopic application of laser energy more than 20 years ago and since then has created a broad range of indications for laser use.

Aided by advances in fiberoptics, the laser has already made a substantial contribution toward minimally invasive operative technique. However, progress will not stop there. Laser techniques will advance to the ultrastructural level and one day will enable surgeons to carry out procedures that can scarcely be imagined today.

Appendix

Instrumentation

Laser instrumentation consists of the laser unit, the delivery system (usually quartz fibers, with CO_2 lasers requiring an articulated-arm mirror system), and special handpieces or endoscopes and endoscopic attachments. All endoscope manufacturers have made their instruments compatible with surgical lasers; this applies to contact and noncontact techniques as well as interstitial laser application. Some examples are shown in the figures below.

Laser Manufacturers

- Aesculap-Meditec GmbH, Medical Laser Systems, Postfach 1, Am Ruhstein 7, D-90562 Heroldsberg, Germany
- Baasel Lasertech, Petersbrunner Strasse lb, D-82319 Starnberg, Germany
- Dornier Medizintechnik GmbH, Industriestrasse 15, D-82110 Germering, Germany
- Heraeus Instruments GmbH, Postfach 15 63, Heraeusstraße 12–14, D-63450 Hanau, Germany
- Jenoptik Technologie GmbH, D-07739 Jena, Germany
- Sharplan Lasers GmbH, Am Lohmühlbach 12a, D-85356 Freising, Germany
- Technolas Laser Technik GmbH, Lochhamer Schlag 19, D-82166 Gräfelfing bei München, Germany

Endoscope Manufacturers

- Karl Storz GmbH & Co., Postfach 230, D-78503 Tuttlingen, Germany
- Olympus Winter & Ibe GmbH, Kuehnstraße 61, D-22045 Hamburg, Germany
- Richard Wolf GmbH, Postfach 11 64–65, D-76434 Knittlingen, Germany

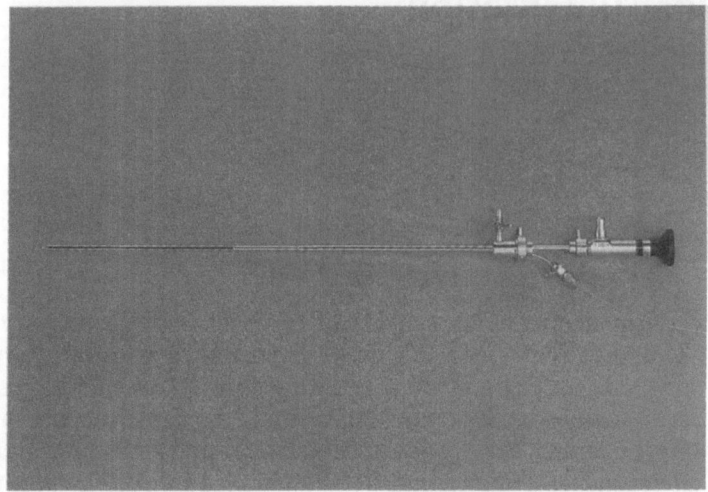

Fig. A1. Laser ureterorenoscope

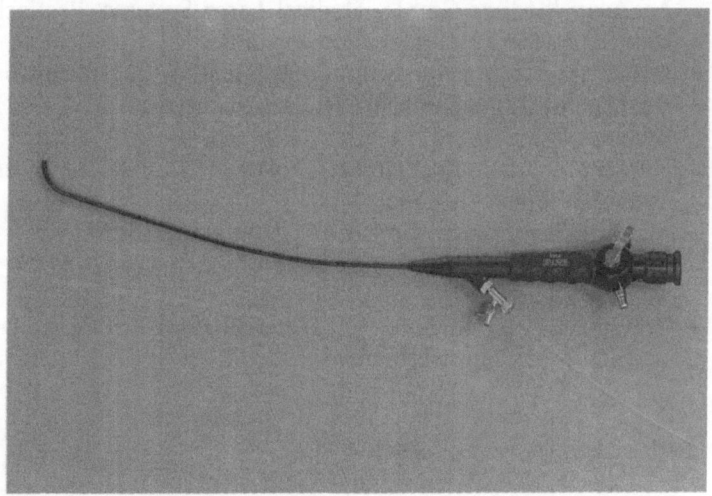

Fig. A2. Flexible laser cystoscope

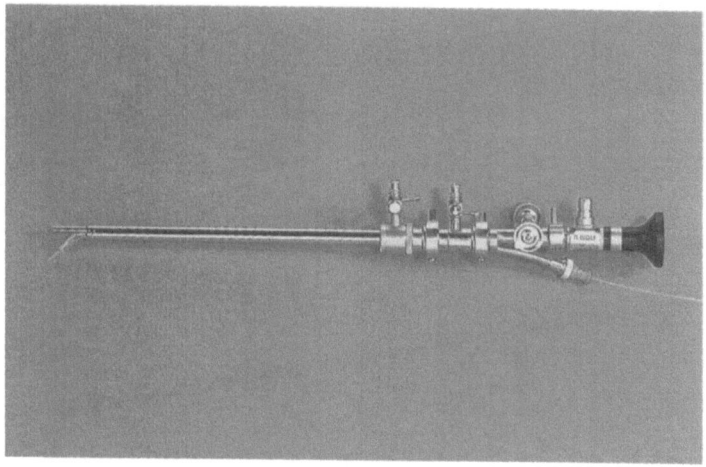

Fig. A3. Percutaneous laser nephroscope (Storz)

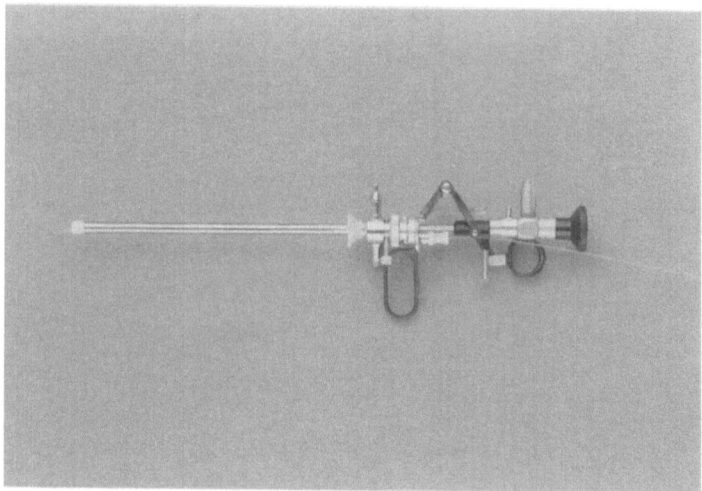

Fig. B1. Laser resectoscope with clamp mechanism for the laser fiber and a universal sheath that allows use of a laser fiber or cutting loop

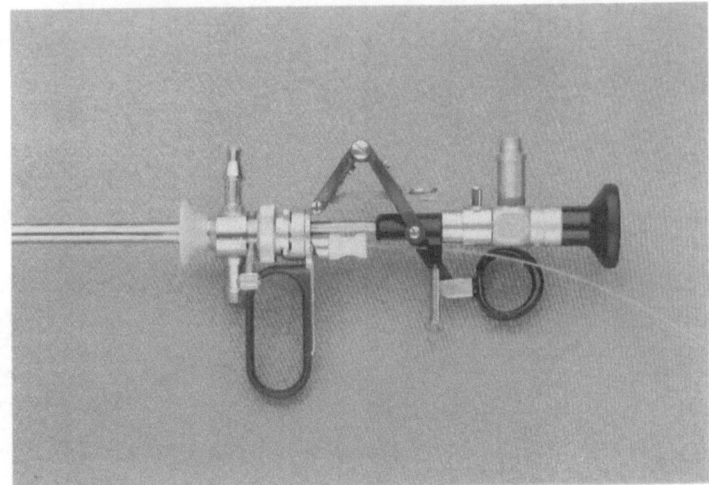

Fig. B2. Laser resectoscope (close-up view)

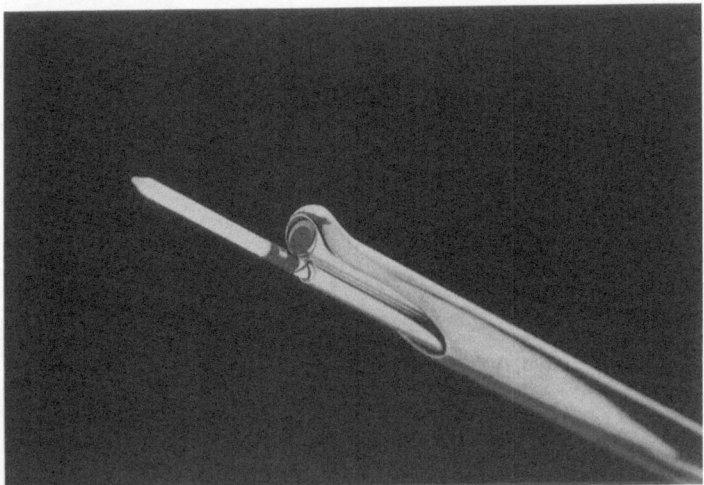

Fig. C. Tip of a cystoscope with special attachment for interstitial laser coagulation of the prostate (designed by Muschter)

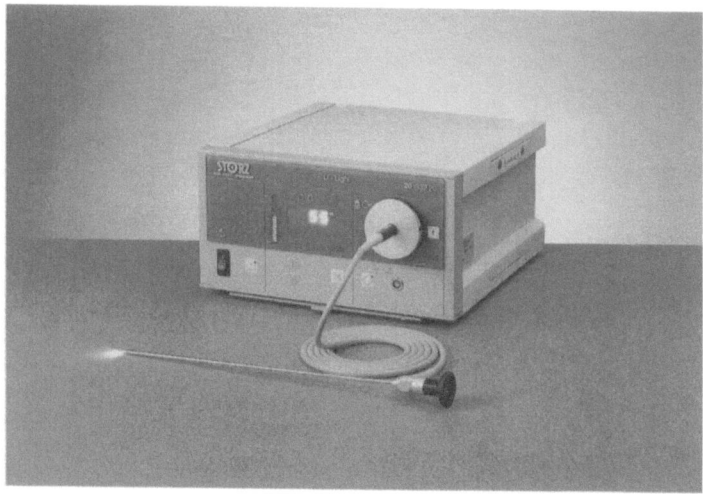

Fig. D1. D light system

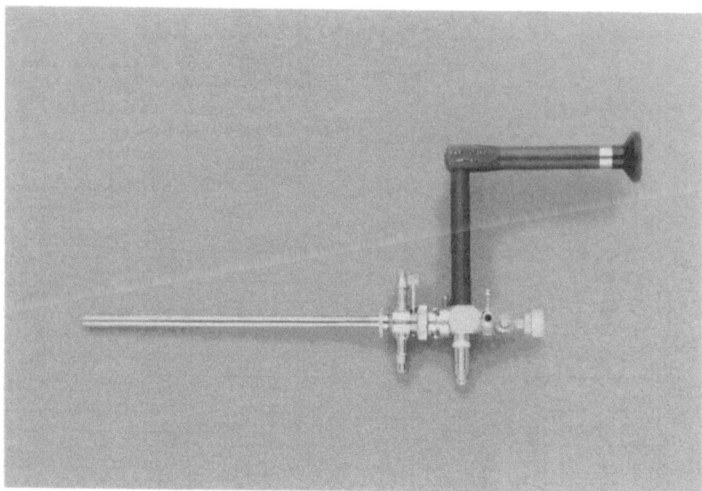

Fig. D2. Laser nephroscope

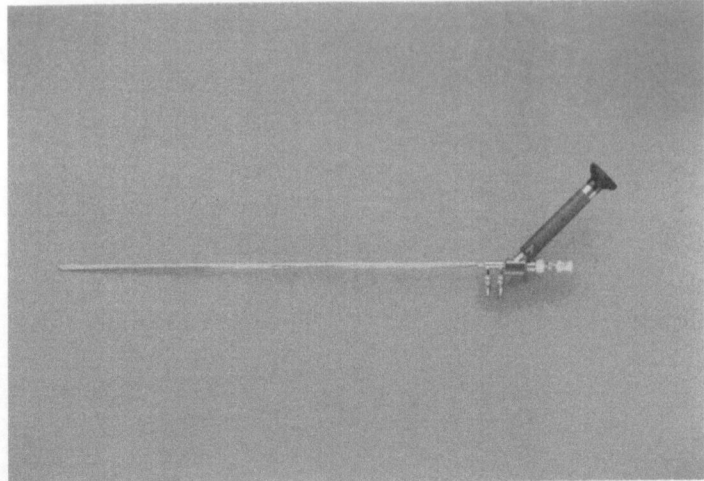

Fig. D3. Laser ureteroscope

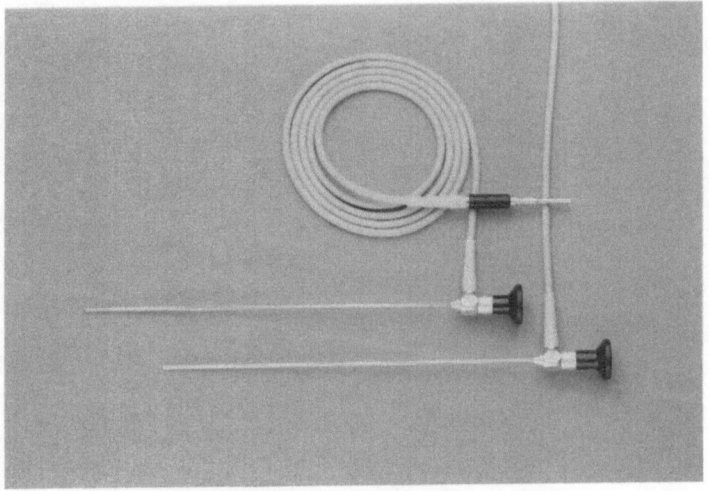

Fig. D4. Optics with built-in fiberoptic cable

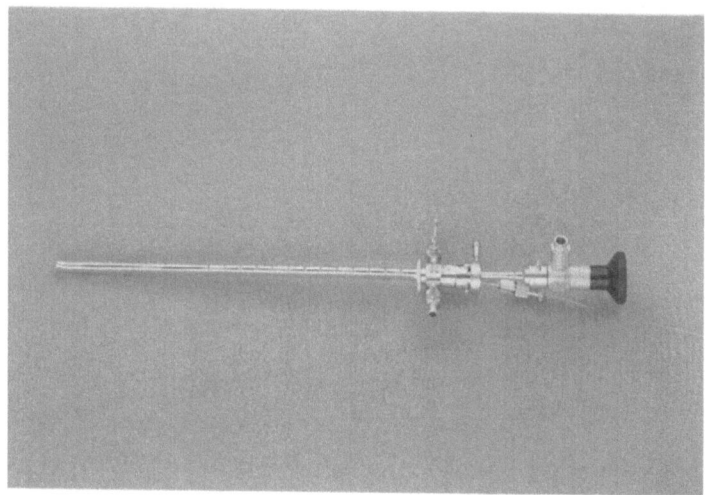

Fig. D5. Laser urethrocystoscope

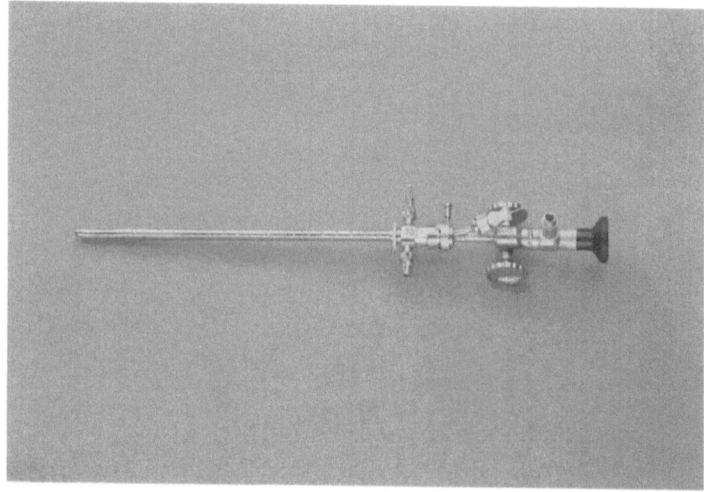

Fig. H1. Laser endoscope with up to 90° angulation of the laser fiber (overall view)

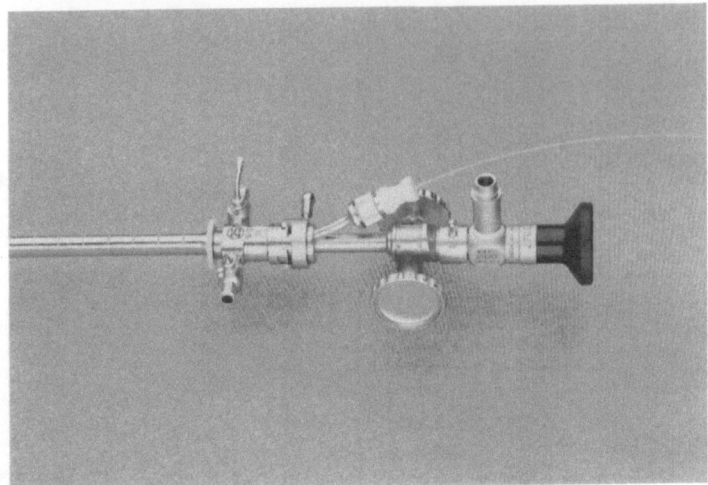

Fig. H2. Close-up view of the endoscope and laser fiber channel

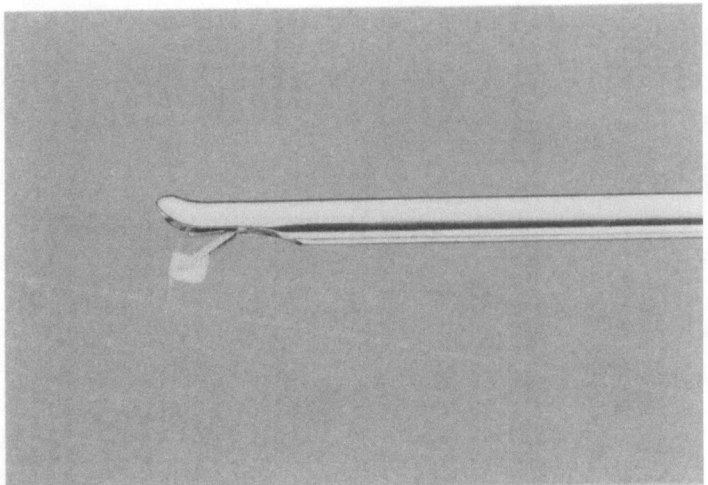

Fig. H3. Endoscope with 80° angulation of the laser fiber tip

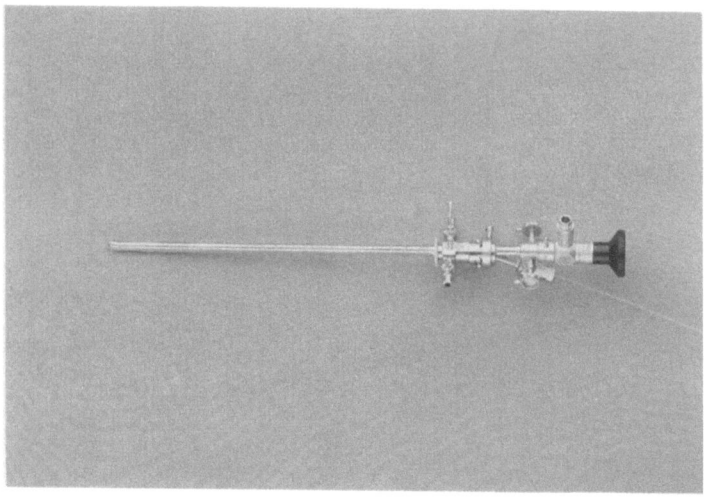

Fig. I1. Laser endoscope (overall view). Instruments I 1–I 3 can be used with side-firing laser probes or with interstitial probes for treating prostatic hyperplasia

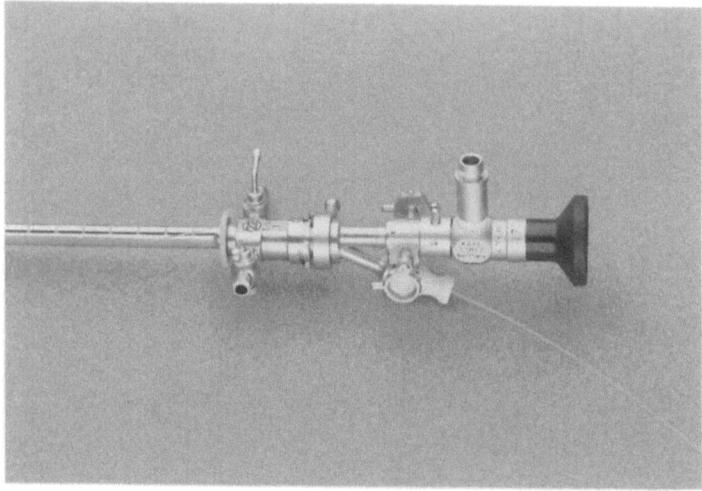

Fig. I2. Endoscope and laser channel (close-up view)

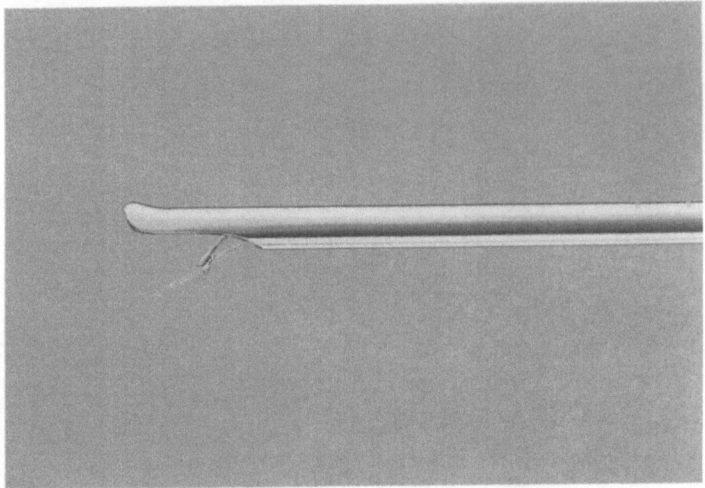

Fig. I3. Endoscope tip with Albarran system for 30°–40° deflection of the laser fiber

Subject Index

ablation 21
absorption 3, 4
acoustic shock waves 30
acoustoontic modulator functions 13
acupuncture 24
alexandrite laser 23, 132, 135
American National Standard Institute 34
5-aminolevulinic acid (ALA) 120
- hydrochloride solutions 49
amplification
- light 3
- microwave 3
argon lasers 16, 65, 127
- specific medical applications 21
aromatic hydrocarbons, heavy exposure 83
articulated-arm mirror system 141
articulating mirrors 18
avalanche breakdown 30

balanitis xerotica obliterans 56
bilevel system 6
biological tissues and laser energy 19–24
- biological effects 22–24
- - nonthermal effects 23, 24
- - - "cold vaporization" 23
- - - photoablation 23
- - - photochemical effects 23
- - - photodisruption 23
- - thermal effects 22
- - - burning 23
- - - carbonization 23
- - - excavation 23
- - - photocoagulation 22
- - - photothermal cutting 23
- - - vaporization 23
- electron excitation 19
- energy transfer 19
- induction of oscillation and rotational modes by IR radiation 19
- ionization 19
- laser-tissue interaction 19
- - absorption 19, 20
- - penetration depths 20
- - reflection 19
- - scattering 19, 20
- - transmission 19
bladder 67–76
- contracted 76
- neck 64
- tumor (cancer) 67
- - "Bulky disease" 76
- - D_3 dysplasia 76
- - endoscopic laser treatment with laparoscopic monitoring 68
- - interstitial laser treatment 74
- - line-by-line irradiation 72
- - multiple carcinomas in situ 76
- - operative techniques 70–76
- - photodynamic diagnosis 119–124
- - recurrent superficial 124
- - vessels 72, 73
- wall, temperature distribution 71
- whole-bladder photoirradiation 125
blood, penetration depths 20
Bohr model 5
Bowen's disease 47, 57
burning 23
Buschke-Löwnstein papilloma 47, 56

capillary sealing 22
carbon gas lasers 16
carbonization 23
carcinoma, penile 49, 56–61
cavernous hemangioma 57
CCD Endocam 5370 with Endocolor system 94
cervical intraepithelial neoplasia 47
cirucumcision 50
CO_2 insufflator 94
CO_2 laser 50, 52, 55, 65, 100, 141
- photocoagulation 101

CO_2 laser
- specific medical applications   21
coagulation   21, 22
- CO_2 laser photocoagulation   101
- interstitial laser coagulation (ILC)
   110, 111, 144
- Nd:YAG laser photocoagulation   121
- transurethral laser coagulation
   105–109
coherent light   13
cold knife excision   54
"cold vaporization"   23
color video camera   121
condylomata acuminata   47, 50–52, 57
contact techniques   141
contact tip   18
continuous-wave
- lasers   30
- mode   9
cryosurgery   54
cutaneous horn   56
cutting   21
cystis, interstitial   81
cystoscope with special attachment for
   interstitial laser coagulation   144
cystoscopy
- conventional   121, 122
- fluorescent   121, 122

D light system   145
damping, periodic   13
delivery system   141
diffraction   4
DIN EN 207, 1993   36
DIN EN 60825-1   34
diode laser   104, 105, 109, 110
diodes, semiconductor   9
Dormia basket   134
Dornier Fibertome   110
dose   12
double-balloon catheter   113
dye laser   8, 16, 23, 24, 135
- pulsed   132
- pumped   127
dysplasia, penile   57

Einstein, A.   3, 6
electrocautery   54
electromagnetic
- radiation
- - depth of penetration   29
- - high-frequency   9
- spectrum   4

- waves   4
electron
- excitation   19
- excited   5
- orbital   5
electrosurgical resection   54
emission, stimulated   3
endoscope   141, 149
- manufactures   141
endoscope tip with Albarran system   150
endoscope with 80° angulation of the
   laser fiber tip   148
endoscopic
- applications   18
- attachments   141
energy
- density   12, 30
- excitation   5
entrapment sack   96, 99
equipment safety   39–43
erbium laser   65
erbium:YAG laser   21
erythroplasia of Queyrat   47
European Laser Association (ELA)   40
excavation   23
excimer laser   7, 16, 65
excitation energy   5
excited electron   5
explosion   37
exposure
- limits   31, 32
- - eye   32
- - skin   32
- time   30
eye protection (injuries)   28, 29, 31, 36
- cornea   28, 31
- exposure limits   32
- laser goggles   36
- lens   28
- protective eye filters   36
- retina   28, 31

fiberoptic technology   137
Fibertome   104, 105
fire, risk of   37
fixed-frequency lasers   17
flashlamp-pumped dye laser   135
flexible fiberoptic waveguides   18
flexible laser cystoscope   142
fluorescence, intensity   119
fluorescent cystoscopy   120, 122
5-fluorouracil   54
forceps, optical   137

four-level
- laser   7
- system   7
free-electron laser   8

galium arsenide semiconductor lasers
  16, 24
gas discharge, high-voltage   9
gas lasers   8, 9, 16
genetic engineering   137
genitalia, external   47-61
- condylomata acuminata   47-56
- - contraindications for laser surgery
    55
- - operative techniques   49-53
- - - advantages   54
- - - application   50-53
- - - technical parameters   49, 50
- intraurethral lesions   52
- penile carcinoma   56-61
- - contraindications   61
- - operating technique   58-60
- - recurrence rates   56, 57
- skin lesions
- - flat   52
- - viral   47
German Standard Institute   33
Germany Society for Laser Medicine
  (DGLM)   40, 41
- certification guidelines   40, 41
- certification program   39, 40
- training program   40
giant pulse   13
gold vapor laser   24

heat
- capacity   22
- conduction   22
- convection   22
helium-neon
- aiming beam   50
- laser   16, 16, 24
hematoporphyrin derivate   24, 119
high-frequency electromagnetic radiation   9
high-voltage gas discharge   9
Hofstetter double-balloon catheter   110
holmium laser   21, 104
holmium:YAG laser   21, 65, 104, 105,
  109
human papillomavirus (HPV)
- lesions   47, 49
- typing   49

Hunner's ulcer   81
hyperthermia   21

image intensifier camera   121
immune system stimulation by photodynamic therapy   120
immunological effects   24
Indigo 830
infrared
- emissions   21
- laser scalpels, depth of cut   21
- radiation   28
- - IR-A   29
- - IR-B   29
- - IR-C   29
instrumentation   141-150
intensity   12
interference   4
internal urethrotomy   64
International Electrotechnical Commission, publication 825-I   33
International Prostatic Symptom Score
  103
interstitial
- cystitis   81
- laser
- - application   141
- - coagulation   22

kidney, solitary   83
krypton lasers   16, 122
KTP laser   65, 104, 109

lamina propria   74
laser(s)   3
- alexandrite   23, 132, 135
- area   33
- argon   65, 127
- - specific medical applications   21
- beam, intensity profile   11
- biostimulaton   24
- catheter by *Hofstetter*   132, 134
- classes   34, 35, 37
- CO_2 50, 52, 55, 65, 100
- - specific medical applications   21
- continuous-wave   30
- cystoscope, flexible   142
- diode   104, 105, 109, 110
- dye   8, 23, 24, 135
- endoscope   149
- - with up to 90° angulation   147
- energy application, delivery systems
    18

laser(s)
- energy application, delivery systems
- - articulated-arm mirror system   18
- - fiberoptic deliverry system   18
- erbium   65
- erbium:YAG   21
- excimer   7, 65
- exposure parameters   12
- - dose   12
- - energy (E)   12
- - - density   12
- - intensity   12
- - power (P)   12
- - - density   12, 15
- Fibertome   99
- fixed-frequency   17
- flashlamp-pumped dye   135
- four-level   7
- free-electron   8
- gas   8, 9, 16
- goggles   36
- gold vapor   24
- He-Ne   15, 24
- holmium   21, 104
- holmium:YAG   21, 65, 104, 105, 109
- KTP   65, 104, 109
- light, properties   13-16
- - beam
- - - diameter   15
- - - divergence   15
- - coherence   13-15
- - - spatial   14
- - - temporal   14
- - monochromaticity   13-15
- - power density   15
- liquid   16
- Lithognost   131, 132
- lithotripsy   131-135
- - advantages   132
- - contraindications   135
- - extracorporeal shock wave (ESWL)
  131
- - indications   131, 132
- - instrumentation   135
- - operative technique   131-135
- - ureteral stones   131
- - ureterscopic   131
- M-locked   30
- manufactures   141
- microbeam   137
- mode-locked   13
- Nd:YAG   22, 50-52, 55, 60, 61, 64, 65,
  74, 79, 81, 104, 105, 109, 110, 132, 135
- - pulsed   135

- - specific medical applications   21
- nephroscope   143, 145
- nitrogen   24
- physics   3-24
- - emission
- - - spontaneous   5
- - - stimulated   5, 6
- - physical principles   4-7
- - wave particle duality   4
- prostatectomy   106
- pulsed   30
- - dye   132
- pumped dye   127
- Q-switched   30
- radiation, physical units   12
- resectoscope   143, 144
- ruby   7
- safety officer   39-41, 43
- scalpels, infrared, depth of cut   21
- semiconductor   7-9, 15, 16
- smoke   37
- solid-state   8, 9, 16
- system(s)
- - for medicine   16
- - operational parameters   17, 18
- - - spectral parameters   17
- - - temporal parameters   17
- - physical components   7-12
- - - lasing medium   7, 8, 10
- - - oscilator   9, 10
- - - pump source   7, 8
- - - resonator   7
- - for urethrotomy   65
- three-level   7
- tunable   17
- unit   141
- ureterorenoscope   142
- ureteroscope   146
- urethrocystoscope   147
- UV-emitting excimer   23
- x-ray   137
laser-induced plasma   23
leukoplakia   47, 56
lichen sclerosus et atrophicus   47
light amplification   3
liquid lasers   16
lithium niobate   17
lithoclast   132
Lithognost   131, 132, 135
lithotomy position   107
long-wave region   28
lymphomas   57
lymphorrhea   97

M-locked lasers 30
Maiman, T. 3
maser 3
McBurney point 96
Medical Equipment Code (MedGV)
    39–42
medical lasers 16
Medilas 4060 N 99
metastable level 6, 13
microwave amplification 3
minimally invasive operative technique
    137
mode locking 13
mode-locked laser 13
modulation cell 13
molecular biology 137
molluscum contagiosum 49
Multiscope 76

n-region 9
Nd:YAG Fibertome 65
Nd:YAG laser 16, 22, 50–52, 55, 60, 61,
    64, 65, 74, 79, 81,104, 105, 109, 110,
    132, 135
– photocoagulation 121
– pulsed 135
– specific medical applications 21
nephroscope, flexible 91
Nesbit technique 104
nitrogen laser 24
noncontact techniques 141

optical forceps 137
optics with built-in fiberoptic cable 146
orbital electron 5
oxalate monohydrate stones 135

p-region 9
Paget's disease 56
particle (corpuscular) model 4
pelvic lymph node status 93
pelvic lymphadenectomy, laparoscopic
    93–99
– operative technique 94–99
– – advantages 98
– – complication rate 98
– – contraindication 99
– – disadvantages 98, 99
– – instrumentation 99
penetration depth 20
– elecromagnetic radiation 29
penile
– carcinoma 49, 56–61

– intraepithelial neoplasia 47
periodic damping 13
phenacetin abuse 83
photoablation 23
photochemical effects 23, 30
photocoagulation (*see also* coagula-
    tion) 22
photodisruption 23
– of molecular structures 137
photodynamic
– diagnosis (PDD) 24, 55, 119–124
– – advantages and disadvantages 123
– – contraindications 123
– – equipment 123
– – – biopsy forceps 124
– – – documentation 124
– – – endoscope 124
– – – excitation fiber 124
– – – light source 123
– – – photosensitizing agent 123
– – indication 121
– – technique 121
– effect 119
– therapy (PDT) 119
– – advantages 125, 126
– – catheter 128
– – contraindications 127
– – disadvantages 127
– – dosimetry 128
– – equipment 127
– – exposure times 126
– – fluorescent cystoscopy 120
– – indications 124
– – photosensitizer 119, 120, 125, 127
– – – Photofrin 120, 125, 127
– – – Photosan-3 120, 125, 127
– – – porphyrin 119
– – stimulation of immune system 120
– – technique 125–128
– – tissue autofluorescence,
    suppression 120
– – transfer of energy 120
Photofrin 120, 125
photon
– absorption 5
– emission 4, 5
– – spontaneous 6
– – stimulated 6
– energy 4
Photosan-3 120, 125
photosensitizer 119, 120
photothermal cutting 23
Planck's constant 4

plasma, laser-induced   23
pn junction   9
pneumoperitoneum   94
podophyllin   54
podophyllotoxin   54
population inversion   6, 13
porphyrin(s)
- monomers   121
- photosensitizers   119
- synthetic   125
power density   12, 30
premalignant lesions   47
prostate, benign prostatic hyperplasia
    102-114
- nomenclature of laser treatments   103
- operation technique   104-111
- - advantages and disadvantages   113,
    114
- - contraindications   114
- - interstitial laser coagulation (ILC)
    110, 111
- - percutaneous transperineal
    approach   111
- - transrectal ultrasound guidance
    111
- - transurethral
- - - approach   110, 111
- - - contact laser vaporization   105
- - - laser ablation/laser vaporization
    109
- - - laser coagulation   105-109
- - - laser incision   104
- - - laser resection (TURP)   104
- - - ultrasound-giuded laser-induced
    prostatctomy   106
- - visual/endoscopic laser ablation   107
- periurethral   105
prostatectomy, laser   106
prostatic carcinoma   114
protective eye filters   36
protein denaturation   22
protoporphyrin IX   121
pulse duration   30
pulsed lasers   30, 132
pyelocaliceal tumors   88-92
- operative techniques   89, 90
- - approaches for laser surgery   90
- - instrumentation   91
- - - lower caliceal groups   90
- - - middle caliceal group   90
- - ureteroscopic approach   90

Q-switched lasers   30
Q-switching   12, 13
quality of life index   103
quantum energy   6
quartz fibers   141
Queyrat's erythroplasia   56, 57

radiation
- area   12
- source   31
- time   12
radio waves   4
Raman spectroscopy   137
reflection   19
refractive index   18
renal
- failure   83
- transplant recipients   83
residual urine, ultrasound determina-
    tion   103
Rhodamine XG   135
Roentgen   3
ruby
- cristal   3, 4
- laser   7

safeguards   27
safety aspects, laser surgery   27-38
- biological hazards   27
- chemical hazards   31
- - protection   37
- electrical hazards   27
- explosion   37
- exposure time   30, 32
- - eye   32
- - skin   32
- eye protections   28, 36
- fire, risk   37
- laser safety officer   39
- patient protection   37
- safety measures   35
- - equipment safety   35, 39-43
- - organizational measures   35
- smoke   37
- technical hazards   31
- - exposure limits   31, 32
- - maximum permissible exposure
    31, 32
- technical standards   33, 34
- thermal injuries   28
- user certification   39-43
scattering   3, 4, 19, 20
Schistosoma haematobium   77

- life cycle   78
schistosomal
- lesions   81
- tubercles   79
Schistosomiasis, urinary   77–82
- cytoscopic findings   79
- late complications   79
- operative techniques   80
- - contraindications   81
semiconductor
- diodes   9
- lasers   7–9, 15, 16
Semm technique   96
shock waves   30
short-wave region   28
skin
- exposure limits   32
- lesions   28
solid-state laser   8, 9, 16
solitary kidney   83
Spanish collar   71, 73
sperm granulomas   101
stones, oxalate monohydrate stones
   135
submucous ulcer   81

technical standards   33, 34
TEM_{00} mode   15
temperature
- critical   22
- peak   22
thermal
- expansion   30
- injuries   28
- relaxation time   22
three-level
- laser   7
- model   7
tissue autofluorescence, suppression
   120
transmission   19
transrectal ultrasound   103
transverse electromagnetic modes   11,
   12
trichloroacetic acid   54
trilevel-energy laser   7
trocar needle   111
tumor capillary system, disruption by
   PDT   120
tumor-specific photosensitizers   24
tunable lasers   17
two-level scheme   6

ulcer, submucous   81
ultrasound determination of residual
   urine   103
ureteral
- stones (*see also* lithotripsy)   131–135
- tumors   83–88
- - contraindications for laser
   treatment   83
- - distribution   85
- - indications for laser treatment   83
- - location   85
- - operative technique   83
- - - instrumentation   88
ureterorenoscopy   132
ureteroscopy   83
urethra   52, 62–66
- dilatation   64
- urethral strictures   62, 64
- - etiology   62
- - operative technique   63–65
- - - advantages   64
- - - contraindications   65
- - instrumentation   65
- Wall stent implantation   65
urethroscopy   49
urethrotomy
- distal laser   66
- internal   64
- laser systems for   65
uroflowmetry   103
urogenital tract
- female   48
- male   48
user certification   39–43
UV
- illumination   121
- laser   121
- light   121
- radiation   28
- - UV-A   28
- - UV-B   28
- - UV-C   28
UV-emitting excimer lasers   23

vaporization   21, 23, 30
vasovasostomy, laser-assisted   100–102
- laser welding   101
- microsurgical   100
- operative technique   101
Veress needle   94
videoendoscope   96
viral vectors   137

water, penetration depths   20
wave(s)   4
– electromagnetic   4
– frequency   4
– length   4, 28
– model   4
– velocity   4

wavefront   3
white light   122

x-ray lasers   137
x-rays   4

Z incision   96